Praise for
Validation Techniques for Dementia Care

"This book gives family members, friends, and others the keys to unlock the doors to continued relationships and opportunities for positive interactions with loved ones. Ms. de Klerk-Rubin presents the principles of Validation, gives meaningful guidance in negotiating the role of caregiver, provides techniques and approaches that have been proven to be useful, and gives excellent examples in the form of stories to guide application. An important contribution to the caregiving literature."

—Harvey L. Sterns, Ph.D., Director, Institute for Life-Span Development and Gerontology and Professor of Psychology, The University of Akron; Research Professor of Gerontology, Northeastern Ohio Universities College of Medicine and College of Pharmacy

"Validation Techniques for Dementia Care . . . uses a combination of narrative and step-by-step guidelines to help readers truly integrate Validation techniques into their interactions with loved ones . . . Reading this book will build mindfulness and empathy in caregivers, teaching them simple methods that can help them explore and support the emotional reality of aging persons and find relevance and meaning in their experiences."

—Peter Whitehouse, M.D., Ph.D., and **Danny George, M.Sc.,** authors of *The Myth of Alzheimer's: What You Aren't Being Told About Today's Most Dreaded Diagnosis*

"How I wish I'd had this book when I was caring for my parents, both suffering from Alzheimer's disease. . . . How much easier it would have been and how much time and heartache it would have saved to have instructions on how to manage the myriad of odd behaviors that occur in those with dementia."

—**Jacqueline Marcell,** author of *Elder Rage*, and host of *Coping with Caregiving*

"As a Validation teacher for 8 years, an administrator for 18 years, and as someone who practices these techniques and leads groups, I can testify that the Validation paradigm is effective, practical, and has a transformative impact. . . . The communication model . . . is really on target; it is an apt psychological and sociological map of the dementia terrain. The techniques listed are skills family members can use to navigate these previously uncharted waters. If your loved one is struggling with dementia, this book is a must-read for you."

—**Scott Averill, J.D.,** CEO, Brookside Retirement Community, Overbrook, Kansas

"Vicki de Klerk-Rubin has penned a powerful complement to Naomi Feil's earlier works. . . . Readers are left with concrete methods and a sense of hope as they toil through very difficult times."

—**Sandy Ransom, R.N., M.S.H.P.,** Director, Texas Long Term Care Institute

Validation Techniques for Dementia Care

Validation Techniques for Dementia Care

The Family Guide to Improving Communication

Vicki de Klerk-Rubin, R.N., M.B.A.

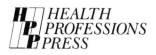
HEALTH
PROFESSIONS
PRESS

Baltimore • London • Sydney

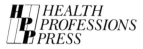

Health Professions Press, Inc.
Post Office Box 10624
Baltimore, Maryland 21285-0624
www.healthpropress.com

Vicki de Klerk-Rubin:
Original manuscript: *"Validation for Family Caregivers"*
© 2006 by Ernst Reinhardt Verlag

Revised licensed English edition: *"Validation Techniques for Dementia Care: The Family Guide to Improving Communication"*
© 2008 by Health Professions Press, Inc.
Title of the German edition 2006: *"Mit dementen Menschen richtig umgehen Validation für Angehörige"*
© 2006 by Ernst Reinhardt Verlag München/Basel
Kemnatenstr. 46, 80639 München, Germany
www.reinhardt-verlag.de

Cover and interior designs by Mindy Dunn. Typeset by Barton Matheson Willse & Worthington, Baltimore, Maryland. Manufactured in the United States of America by Victor Graphics, Baltimore, Maryland.

Library of Congress Cataloging-in-Publication Data
Klerk-Rubin, Vicki de.
  Validation techniques for dementia care : the family guide to improving communication / by Vicki de Klerk-Rubin.
      p. ; cm.
  Includes bibliographical references and index.
  ISBN-13: 978-1-932529-37-1 (pbk.)
  1. Senile dementia—Patients—Care. 2. Caregivers. I. Title.
  [DNLM: 1. Alzheimer Disease—psychology. 2. Alzheimer Disease—therapy. 3. Caregivers—psychology. 4. Communication. 5. Family—psychology. WT 155 K64v 2007]
  RC524.K54 2007
  616.8'31—dc22

                                                    2007035571

British Library of Cataloguing-in-Publication data are available from the British Library.

Contents

About the Author

Vicki de Klerk-Rubin is the European manager of the Validation Training Institute and a certified Validation Master. She is the co-author of the 1992 revision of *Validation: The Feil Method* and the second edition of *The Validation Breakthrough: Simple Techniques for Communicating with People with "Alzheimer's-Type Dementia."* Ms. de Klerk-Rubin holds a bachelor of fine arts from Boston University and a master's of business administration from Fordham University, and is a Dutch-trained registered nurse. Since 1989, Ms. de Klerk-Rubin has given Validation workshops, lectures, and training programs in Austria, Belgium, Denmark, England, Finland, France, Germany, Italy, Japan, Luxemburg, the Netherlands, Sweden, and the United States. She also has worked in numerous nursing facilities in Amsterdam, leading Validation groups and training staff.

Ms. de Klerk-Rubin, a native New Yorker, is married to a Dutch diplomat and has two daughters who were born in Vienna, Austria. Together they have spent the last twenty years living in Amsterdam, Vienna, Bonn, and The Hague.

With thanks to Deb Kunkel and the many family caregivers with whom she works for sharing their personal stories.

My thanks go to Dr. R.J. Peters, Bernice Wollman, and Piet de Klerk for their expertise and efforts to make this a better book.

Introduction

This book is for people who are caring for disoriented very old loved ones. It is for daughters, daughters-in-law, sons, sons-in-laws, husbands, wives, brothers, sisters, friends, neighbors, and other extended "family members." It does not matter whether you are caring for loved ones at home or in an institution, handling all of the care or just a part of it. If your loved one has received a diagnosis of some form of dementia and he or she is in his or her late 70s or older, then this book might help you.

Validation is a method of communicating with and helping very old people with dementia in their final stage of life. The goal is not to make disoriented elderly better but rather to help caregivers to change themselves so that they can enter the personal reality of the person for whom they are caring. Through a caring, empathic relationship, caregivers can reconnect or connect in a new way and give their disoriented relative more ease and pleasure. This is what Validation offers those who are distressed by the pain, effort, and anxiety that come with caring for disoriented elderly. Although Validation is not curative, it has value to the caregiver and the care recipient. When a caregiver has an intimate conversation, shares a laugh or a tear, or finally understands behavior that has seemed bizarre, it can be profoundly rewarding. Caregivers experience a feeling of relief when they do not need to fight or struggle to change their relative. Their self-respect increases as they feel more competent. Validation brings relief to and honors the humanity of the elderly. They benefit from less stress and from feeling accepted and valued for who they are now. Encouraged to communicate about issues that matter to them, they can keep connected to you instead of withdrawing further into themselves.

Validation does not require a lot of time, but it does ask a great deal from its practitioners. To practice Validation, you must be honest with yourself, face your own feelings, be able to set those feelings aside for a short time, and be willing to deal openly with the feelings of your relative. Not everyone wants to take these steps. It could be that after looking through this book you decide that Validation may be right for your relative but not something that you want to do. However, even a passive understanding of the Validation theories and goals can influence your attitude toward your relative and your situation and improve the way you respond to him or her. Also, if Validation is incorporated into the professional care of a loved one, then it is of value to family members and to their loved one to understand the basic principles.

This book will not teach you everything about Validation but will give you enough to make a start, and perhaps that will be enough to open up a whole new way of being with your disoriented relative. Part I starts with a basic primer in Validation principles and theory. Not all theory is discussed but enough to lead you to form realistic goals and support a basic emotional posture. Then comes a look at the relevance of and the meaning behind the behavior of disoriented very old people. This is followed in Part II by a step-by-step description of how you can use the Validation method with your disoriented relative. Part III gives several typical scenarios between family members and disoriented relatives and how Validation was used in each case. The commentary that follows each scenario is meant to give you specific ways of handling difficult situations.

The Validation method was created by Naomi Feil (1932), an American gerontologist. She found that the methods she was taught did not work in practice. She began to experiment, and through trial and error came up with a number of ideas, theories, and techniques that over time she formed into a cohesive method. Today, Validation is practiced in hospitals, in nursing facilities, and by community care workers in North America, Europe, Australia, and Japan. Naomi Feil's books *Validation: The Feil Method* (1982, 1989, 2003) and *The Validation Breakthrough* (1993, 2002) both are still in wide distribution and have been translated into nine languages. Introductory videos are available in several languages and are used by many institutions and schools to sensitize and train staff in this humanistic way of working with individuals with dementia of the Alzheimer's type. Naomi Feil has appeared numerous times on television and radio in the United States, Europe, and Japan; 15,000 professional and lay people attend her workshops each year. For more than 15 years, the Validation Training Institute has offered training and certification in the method, following international quality standards. Certification is recognized by many professional organizations and governments. The Validation Training Institute works with an international network of Authorized Validation Organizations. These are listed in Appendix 4 and can be contacted directly for further information, assistance, training possibilities, or the names of Validation practitioners in your area.

Part I

Understanding What Happens to the Disoriented Very Old

Alzheimer's, Dementia, Disorientation: What's in a Name?

One of the greatest challenges to the health care system is the growing number of elderly people with some form of dementia. Not only is the population growing older than ever before, but also a greater number of people are older than 65 years. From 1955 to 2004, the average life span increased from 69.7 years to 77.8 years (National Center for Health Statistics). The most significant factors for this increase in life span are better and more accessible medical care, improved medical technology, and healthful lifestyle choices. In 1950, significant numbers of people died of tuberculosis and

For simplicity, I have chosen to use the female pronoun throughout this book. Everything is, of course, equally applicable for men.

pneumonia. Today, those causes of death do not often occur. Society now has a new and significant segment of the population: those who are older than 80 years. Every sector of society is struggling to understand and deal with the special needs of people in this stage of life.

Concurrent to this shift in the population is a rise in the number of people who receive a diagnosis of Alzheimer's-related dementias: In 2007 in the United States, 5.1 million people have received a diagnosis of Alzheimer's-related dementia. This number is expected to increase to 13.2 million by 2050. What does that mean? Is it that the disease is spreading? Are simply more people developing Alzheimer's disease? Could it be that the diagnosis is more easily made with new technology and so more people are receiving a correct diagnosis, or has the term *Alzheimer's disease* changed so that more people with similar symptoms fit under that diagnosis?

Mrs. D was 51 years of age when she began forgetting normal, everyday things. Also, she suspected her husband of having affairs and became extremely jealous. There was no cause for this in reality, but still she raged at him. She would get lost in her own apartment and carried things around without a purpose and hid them. Sometimes she thought that she would be murdered and would scream. It was at this point that she was committed to an institution. There, her behavior changed; she became helpless and confused about time and about where she was. She would carry parts of her bed around, would call for her husband and daughter, and had auditory hallucinations. She deteriorated continuously until her death 4.5 years later. At the end, she lay in a fetal position, totally withdrawn and unresponsive to her environment. She died at age 55. This happened 100 years ago.

Alois Alzheimer was a German pathologist, who was born in Marktbreit, Bavaria, in 1864. Dr. Alzheimer worked in the institution where Mrs. D had spent her last years and he developed new materials and techniques for examining brain cells. His goal was to find the abnormal structures in the brain that correlated with different neurological and psychiatric illnesses. Over 15 years, with his colleagues Dr. Nissl and Dr. Kraepelin, he published a six-volume encyclopedia, *Histologic and Histopathologic Studies of the Cerebral Cortex* (Alzheimer & Nissl, 1904–1918). In 1906, Dr. Alzheimer first presented his research on the disease that would be named after him (Alzheimer and Nissl). Dr. Alzheimer performed the autopsy on Mrs. D, and he discovered something new. The brain of Mrs. D showed "remarkable changes of the neurofibrillae (parts of nerve cells in the brain). In place of a normal cell, one or several fibrillae were prominent by their thickness and ability to take on stain. . . . The nucleus and the cell disintegrated; subsequently, only a mass of fibrillae showed the site of a ganglion cell. . . . Over the entire brain, and especially in the upper layers, miliary centers appeared, which were caused by an unusual substance. . . . The glia became fibrous, and many glia cells showed fatty deposits . . . apparently we are dealing with an unidentified illness." The fatty deposits have come to be known as *plaques* and the mass of fibers as *tangles*. These are the primary physical symptoms of Alzheimer's disease.

The illustration that follows shows a healthy neuron (nerve cell found in the brain) compared to a neuron with Alzheimer's plaques and tangles. The brain is made up of neurons (nerve cells), which regulate everything that people do, from the basic body functions (e.g., breathing, heart beat, metabolic functions), to automatic behavior (e.g., eye blinking), to conscious behavior (e.g., walking to the store to buy a newspaper).

Nearly 100 years after Dr. Alzheimer first published his findings, scientists are closer to understanding and documenting the disease process. This field is dynamic, research is ongoing, and new information is published on a regular basis. It is not the purpose of this book to provide readers with technical information about Alzheimer's disease. This information can be found in a number of sources, which are listed at the end of this book. What has not progressed far is the process of diagnosis. Still, accurate diagnosis is done only after death, by autopsy and looking at the condition of

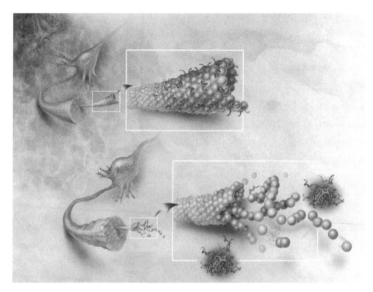

A healthy neuron and a neuron with Alzheimer's plaques and tangles.

the brain. In 2001, scientists at the University of California, Los Angeles were making progress with a new method of identifying so-called Alzheimer's plaques, or amyloid plaques, using a chemical marker called FDDNP. This tracer molecule attaches itself to the plaques and then can be seen on a positron emission tomography (PET) scan. This could prove to be an important diagnostic tool in the future. Even then, there often are surprises. Studies have shown that some people who were oriented until their deaths showed advanced deterioration in their brain on autopsy; some people who were totally disoriented had relatively little brain deterioration. Clearly, other factors are involved in determining whether a person becomes disoriented in late life, which brings us to the next question: What is Alzheimer's disease, and how is that term used? The term *Alzheimer's disease* often is used as an umbrella term to cover many people who have some form of dementia. *Dementia* is itself a general term to describe a syndrome, or series of symptoms. Most psychiatric textbooks define dementia as a chronic, progressive decline in cognitive functions as a result of physiological reasons. One can see deterioration of memory, thinking, orientation, comprehension, calculation, learning ability, use of language, and judgment. There is a big difference between dementia and a delirium. Although often associated with alcohol abuse, a *delirium* is any deterioration in cognitive functions (the same functions as for dementia) that occurs within a short period of time. The reason that it is important to know the difference between dementia and a delirium is because sometimes people's illness is misdiagnosed. An example of this is when a very old person has a medical emergency (e.g., a broken hip), is brought to the hospital, and becomes disoriented. Before one can make a diagnosis of dementia, one has to know whether the disoriented behavior was present before the medical emergency. Often, people become disoriented, agitated, emotionally expressive, or depressed when confronted with a traumatic situation. It is a reaction to an unusual occurrence, not deterioration of the brain, that is behind the behavior. Emergency personnel are not specially trained to recognize the difference, and often a patient is labeled as having dementia when in fact that is not the case. There are some signs that emergency personnel are recognizing this as a problem, and geriatric specialists are being used more for consultations in emergency departments to prevent this sort of misdiagnosis.

An elderly person who has a small stroke also sometimes receives a misdiagnosis. One of the symptoms of a stroke is strange behavior or delirium. This generally is acute, meaning that it begins immediately after the event (rather than gradually getting worse) and tends to get better over time. Mini-strokes often happen in such a way that they do not get recognized and go undiagnosed. A person wakes up in the morning feeling strangely, a bit weak, and confused. It is easy enough to chalk it up to a virus or not enough sleep or a bad day. Often the symptoms are treated without looking at the entire picture. Treatment with psychotropic drugs or even heavy dosages of antibiotics can cause even more disorientation. The cycle of symptoms–treatment–symptoms–treatment can lead to deeper and deeper withdrawal.

There are many different reasons for dementia. The following list identifies various forms (DSM IV & ICD-10; World Health Organization); many of the symptoms are similar:

- Alzheimer's disease

- Dementia of the Alzheimer's Type (DAT)

- Alcoholic dementia (Korsakoff's syndrome)

- Multi-infarct dementia, also known as vascular dementia

- Huntington's disease

- Parkinson's disease

- Pick's disease

- HIV

- Substance-induced persisting dementia (as a result of long-term drug abuse or a reaction to a medication or toxin; many elderly people have extreme reactions to medications or are highly sensitive to medications—what would be considered an appropriate dosage for a middle-aged person would cause an "intoxication" in older people)

- Brain injuries or tumors

- Endocrine conditions (e.g., hypothyroidism, hypercalcemia, hypoglycemia)

- Immune disorders (e.g., polymyalgia rheumatica, systemic lupus erythematosus)

- Neurological conditions (e.g., multiple sclerosis)

Most of these illnesses or conditions can be diagnosed with specific testing, such as blood tests, urinalysis, chest x-ray, electrocardiogram, brain imaging (computed tomography [CT] scan or magnetic resonance imaging [MRI] scan). The term *Alzheimer's disease* refers to a very specific illness, one that can be diagnosed only by eliminating all other possibilities. It is a diagnosis that is made by exclusion. The disease has a gradual beginning, starting in one's 40s, 50s, or 60s, and a continuing decline. Experienced and observant professionals who work with disoriented elderly on a daily basis often can see the difference between a person with Alzheimer's disease and a person with Korsakoff's syndrome, for example, by physical characteristics, such as the way of walking, holding the head, making eye contact, facial expression, and the use of speech.

Many families first go to their family doctor with the suspicion that something is wrong with their relative and the fear that it could be Alzheimer's disease. Doctors generally perform the following three assessments:

- Take a personal medical history
- Do a physical examination and get laboratory tests
- Evaluate the mental status using what is known as the Mini-Mental State Examination

Often, family caregivers are questioned about changes that they have noticed, symptoms that worried them, the daily routine, whether the symptoms have remained constant or grown worse over time, and whether the symptoms are interfering with daily activities. The doctor also may ask about the family member's personal medical history; family medical history, including mental illness and dementia; the person's social and cultural background; and all information about prescription and over-the-counter medications, including vitamins, minerals, and herbal preparations that the person is taking.

The physical examination and laboratory testing should include the following:

- A physical examination to look for medical illnesses, such as congestive heart failure or diabetes, that may contribute to cognitive impairment

- A neurological examination to identify signs of Parkinson's disease, stroke, tumor, or other medical conditions that may affect memory and thinking
- A head and brain scan, by CT scan or MRI scan, to look for shrinkage (atrophy) of memory structures, stroke, or fluid in the brain (hydrocephalus)
- Blood and urine tests to pinpoint any possible thyroid problems, anemia, medication imbalances, or infections
- An electrocardiogram, which records the electrical activity of the heart
- A chest X-ray

The Mini-Mental State Examination is a series of questions plus a few written tests that try to determine the person's

- Awareness of time and place
- Memory problems
- Ability to do simple calculations, write, and draw

In some cases, the person might be referred to a neurologist or a specialist in psychogerontology for further testing.

There is no cure for Alzheimer's disease. Many medications on the market may slow the degenerative process and in fact lengthen the life span of people with Alzheimer's disease. The first Alzheimer's patient, Mrs. D, lived 4.5 years after being placed in a mental hospital for her condition. Now, there may be 10 years between diagnosis and the final stages of the disease.

Alzheimer's disease is sometimes called Dementia of the Alzheimer's Type (DAT) with early onset. Another condition that often is mistaken for Alzheimer's disease is what is known as DAT with late onset. These two conditions share many of the same symptoms, but there are significant differences (see sidebar).

Dementia of the Alzheimer's Type (DAT)

DAT with late onset

Disorientation begins much later in life, usually past 80 years of age.

Disorientation does not always progress or lead to death.

Speech can remain intact.

Gait (way of walking) can be dance-like, purposeful, dreamy, aimless, and so forth.

Facial expression is varied and often filled with emotions.

Expression of emotion increases with disorientation.

DAT with early onset/Alzheimer's disease

Disorientation begins early, usually late 50s through 70s.

Disorientation is progressive and leads to death.

Speech deteriorates quickly; people with Alzheimer's disease often quickly lose the ability to communicate verbally.

People with Alzheimer's disease often walk stiffly, robot-like, and without purpose.

People with Alzheimer's disease often have a mask-like expression and do not often express emotion in later stages.

People with Alzheimer's disease have less emotional expression as the disease progresses.

DAT with late onset is the population that Naomi Feil, the developer of Validation, calls the disoriented old-old. She chose the word *disoriented* for a reason. *Dementia* comes from the Latin *de,* meaning "away from," and *mens,* meaning "mind." Feil believes that disoriented old-old are not "away from their minds" or "mindless" but rather more *in their minds* in the sense that they enter into a personal reality that often is quite different from the commonly accepted reality. Of course *reality* is based on personal perceptions. Everyone sees the world differently, but there is an accepted norm that is based on broad socially accepted beliefs and values. Validation theory (which is described in great detail later) attributes disorientation to the inability of people to handle the physical, social, and psychological losses that build up as they age. This inability to cope creates isolation, withdrawal, and a return to the past. The past becomes more important and more vibrant than the present. It is more filled with meaning, comfort, or urgency. In other words, today's weather or politics has less meaning to many very old people than what happened to them during World War II, for example, so personal experiences from the past become the present.

What is important for family members to realize is that there is a great difference between people with early-onset Alzheimer's disease and the disoriented old-old (DAT with late onset). Disorientation stems from a totally different source. Despite that a relative may have a diagnosis of "Alzheimer's disease," one should look carefully at how the diagnosis was made and try to determine whether the relative falls into the late-onset or early-onset patterns of behavior. In both cases, Validation can be helpful as a method of communication and relationship building, but it works far better and with more positive results with those who are disoriented old-old.

WHEN IT HAPPENS IN YOUR FAMILY

Most family members are filled with an avalanche of emotions when they hear that their mother, father, partner, friend, or sibling has "Alzheimer's"—relief at finally knowing the cause of the strange behavior, fear of losing the loved one, hopelessness from thinking that it cannot get better, and helplessness from not knowing what to do. At times, family members feel anger, frustration, sorrow, and even despair. Know that this is normal. Know that these are appropriate reactions, and accept them. Be honest with yourself; be kind to yourself. One of the most important principles of Validation is that feelings such as anger, sadness, and pain are relieved when they are expressed. When these feelings are repressed, they get worse. Repressed or swallowed emotions that are never allowed to come out become "emotional ulcers." They fester under the skin, becoming an abscess waiting to burst. You feel better once the "wound is cleaned." Like an ulcerated sore, the proper treatment is to clean the wound regularly and apply a fresh bandage until it is closed. The next step is to leave it open. Scar tissue forms, and it is healed. It will always be different, perhaps more sensitive, perhaps less, maybe discolored or a different texture. In any case, you carry that with you through the rest of your life. Emotional wounds are similar. They need to be cleaned by expression of feelings and then given rest on a regular basis—not just one outburst but often, whenever the emotions build up. Finding others who have had similar experiences to talk to helps. Having someone in your life with whom you can express yourself is terribly important. Some people benefit greatly from some form of counseling, simply to be able to express the feelings in a safe environment. That is the point. That is the first step in your own treatment plan. Take your emotional needs seriously.

Although it may sound like old-fashioned advice, make sure that you are eating well and sleeping enough. Eat well-balanced meals, and keep sugar and caffeine products under control. Make sure you are drinking enough water—at least 1.5 liters per day. Most adults need 7 to 8 hours of sleep each night. If you are running around on 6 hours of sleep, then you may be sleep deprived and less able to cope with things. Do not forget to create moments of peace when you can really relax: 15 minutes in a hot bath or listening to your favorite piece of music could be just the break you need to refresh your energy. If you are off balance, then you cannot help your disoriented relative. Sometimes it may feel as though you are unable to find the time to take care of yourself. If your relative keeps you awake at night, or you feel that your entire day is spent keeping a close eye on her, then it may seem impossible. Appendix 1 offers a few practical tips and ideas for handling such situations. Hopefully, once you begin to use Validation, those moments will occur less frequently and you can handle them with less stress.

The first important and most difficult step for you in handling your feelings is to accept your disoriented loved one as she is now. Whether this person has early- or late-onset DAT does not matter. She cannot be expected to change and go "back to normal." The norm has changed. If you hope and strive to have your relative behave the way you want her to, then you will be disappointed. Your relative will not be helped. If you cannot accept your relative without trying to change her, then you will not be able to work through your own emotions. Instead, you will keep butting your head against a wall of frustration. Validation practitioners accept people just the way they are in the moment and do not try to change them. Acceptance is difficult because, in some ways, it means saying good-bye to the person you love.

Many family members think that it is better if the disoriented person is "brought back to reality." This is not always so. Think about what kind of reality you are wishing on your loved one. It often is a reality in which she has little worth, little to do to keep productive, and little authority or honor. There is nothing strongly holding your relative to the present reality, and there is a great deal of pull from the past. The needs of the elderly are different from the needs of younger people. What you experience as important is not necessarily important to your relative.

Disoriented people often express feelings that have never before been expressed. This can be surprising or even disturbing for family members. Accepting those feelings also can be challenging, especially when they are directed at you. "That is not my father." "He doesn't make sense." "I want to help, but he won't let me." All three of these often-heard phrases reflect difficulty accepting the disoriented relative. That's right; your father is different now. He is not necessarily interested in his role as a father anymore. Other issues and other times of his life are perhaps more important. He feels emotions that are left over from his history. Things that he has bottled up over years come to the surface and demand attention. He expresses those feelings because it hurts him to keep them inside. What you call "help" may in fact not help at all. If you are trying to get your father to behave in a certain way or trying to confront him with his failures, then he will not be appreciative. The best way to help him is to let him express whatever it is that needs to get out.

Family members who care for disoriented loved ones need to learn skills to help themselves. They need to learn how to handle their own feelings so that they do not project them onto the disoriented relative. They need to learn how to clear themselves of feelings, judgments, and worries so that they can see and hear accurately. They need to find support systems because they cannot do it alone. Validation is a method that many find useful because it teaches how to center and how to observe disoriented elderly to understand them, and it offers specific techniques that can be used to communicate with them.

THE PRINCIPLES OF VALIDATION: TOOLS FOR THINKING DIFFERENTLY

Everything that is done in Validation is guided by principles that help you see your disoriented relative in a different light and help you choose the best way to communicate with her. Take time as you read each principle, and think of how you can use each practically.

All People Are Valuable, Including Those Who Are Disoriented

Even though society tends to look down on the elderly and infirm, do not fall into the trap of seeing your relative as less worthwhile. She has lived long and built up a wealth of experience and wisdom. These are important assets. Modern Western society no longer values the wisdom that comes with age. Instead, it values youth and productivity. With this shift in values, we have lost the pleasure of sitting and listening to stories of the past, lost our verbal history,

Wisdom Expressed by Disoriented Elderly
(van Diemen & van de Nieuwegiessen, 1995)

"Good will is the path from me to you."

"It's better to be crazy. Then people don't expect so much."

"I need my mother, and so she's there for me."

"I had a way of thinking, and now it's gone."

"This is the shadow of my life."

"My thoughts are on the other side, here I have nothing."

"I forget things because I think so deeply."

"When I think of the past, then I get lost in my head."

"When you become demented, you don't talk with others, you think with them, you feel with them."

"If you can hear and understand all the unusual things of demented people, then you are on the same wavelength. Other people are on the short wave, they're not open to it."

and taken away one of our greatest sources of knowledge and in-spiration: our elders. A person does not lose that knowledge with the development of disorientation. Often that wisdom is expressed poetically regardless of whether we are listening (see sidebar). Treat disoriented people with respect, and give them honor.

Disoriented Old-Old Should Be Accepted as They Are

The actions of a person who is disoriented, no matter how bizarre, have a very real and important meaning. It is part of a healing process, and it is not helpful to try to change that. This may seem totally opposite to what you feel, have been told, or have learned. You know that you cannot change another person unless that person wants to change. So it is with disoriented elderly: They cannot change. Your goal is to develop a better relationship with this person and to communicate with her, not to change behavior. The first step is simply to accept her as she is. This will make you feel better and eventually lead to a better relationship.

What this also means is that you have to let go. Your mother or father is becoming different from the mother or father whom you knew. This is the first step of saying good-bye, and that can be painful or difficult. Realize that this is your process and very different from what your relative experiences or needs at this moment. Be aware of your desire to have your relative "be like she was" because that would make you feel more comfortable. This is not to denigrate your feelings of loss or your needs, but it simply is not realistic to try to get your relative to adapt to your needs. It will not work, and everyone will feel worse. As mentioned previously, your needs also are important, and you should not forget them, but try to do that in a way that will help yourself as well as your relative. Correcting your relative's behavior or trying to get her to act in a certain way will only create frustration, withdrawal, confusion, angry outbursts, and a slow degeneration to more disorientation.

There Is a Reason Behind the Behavior of Very Old People

As stated in the previous section, the actions of a disoriented person, no matter how bizarre, have a very real and important meaning. This refers only to that category of disoriented very old people who fall into the population that responds best to Validation; that is, people whose disorientation stems from the inability to cope with the physical, psychological, and social losses that come with age. These people are in the final life stage that Feil calls *resolution* and they are preparing for death. Without being aware cognitively, they seem to "focus" on resolving unfinished issues; relieving boredom; reliving pleasurable experiences; and/or retreating from painful, present-day reality. This process is similar to the way adolescents are driven to assert their identity and rebel against authority or the tendency of older people to reflect on the past. This is not a thought-through plan but a primitive drive that is triggered by the stage of life and by the physical and emotional characteristics of the individual. From the older person's perspective, his or her behavior makes sense and has purpose. From a caregiver's perspective, it often is difficult to see the connection between the purpose and the behavior. This is where Validation comes into play and helps. Validation helps family members and caregivers look closely at these connections, explore them, and see them as extremely important, more important than the facts of everyday reality. The caregiver enters into the personal reality of the disoriented person simply to be there with her so that the person is not isolated and can express herself; by doing so, the caregiver understands the disoriented person better and creates a warm, nurturing relationship.

Very Old Disoriented People
Are in the Final Life Stage: Resolution

In Validation theory, very old age is seen as a distinct stage of life with an important life task: to resolve unfinished "business" before death. Everyone has experienced those flashes of memory of events from the past that never were finished and remain slightly uncomfortable—the "I should have's" or "if I had only's." Mistakes that were made, quarrels that were left incomplete, and injustices, fears, or traumas that were never worked through to an acceptable conclusion and that were pushed aside or repressed at the time come back. These are some examples of what is called the unfinished business of very old age. Strong feelings that are associated with these memories rise up once again, and the discomfort of never having finished the issue becomes stronger than the need to push it away. The struggle in the last stage of life is to try to find some degree of resolution and peace. This is very different from what society teaches about very old age. Validation theory holds that very old people have an important task and that we should not only value it but also assist the older person by accompanying her in this task. I use the word *accompany* because one person cannot guide the other, nor lead or push the other, nor take over the task. All that we can do is be there, have empathy, and share the feelings—and that often is enough.

When Recent Memory Fails, Older Adults Try to Restore Balance to Their Lives by Retrieving Earlier Memories

Recent memory deteriorates with age. Recent memory, or short-term memory, is the part of memory that handles information initially before it gets transferred to long-term memory. Examples of this are: remembering names of people to whom you are introduced at a party, what you want to buy at the supermarket, and what you had for breakfast this morning. Examples of long-term memory are: "David blew out my birthday candles at my fourth birthday party," being beat up by the school bully at age 12, and wedding day memories. Long-term memory often is associated with emotional events, and the memories remain vibrant into old-old age. It is easy to imagine that vibrant long-term memories, filled with emotion and importance, would come up more frequently in very old age. It is, as already mentioned, a natural part of this stage of life to review the past and resolve unfinished business. Now add to this that many older adults have deteriorated vision and hearing, which means that information from the surroundings is not as sharp or clear. Awareness of surroundings often is diminished because of deterioration of all of the senses. The present is cloudy and dim; the past is clear and vibrant. The present often is painful, not just physically but more often psychologically: sitting uselessly, not listened to, not valued, bored by the lack of stimulation. If the older adult lives in a nursing or other facility, then she is likely surrounded by disoriented residents, strangers, and staff and may not know where she is. How understandable and easy it is to slip into pleasant memories from long ago. The past becomes a refuge from an unendurable present.

When Eyesight Fails, Older Adults Use the Mind's Eye to See; When Hearing Goes, They Listen to Sounds from the Past

There is a physiological basis for this principle: Every person can stimulate sensory memories simply by thinking about them. Try the following exercise; as you read the sentences, take time before you move on to the next sentence:

- Think about the last time you walked into a bakery and fresh bread was coming out of the oven.

- Think about the taste of a sour lemon drop.

- Think about the sound of your mother's voice.

- Think about the colors of a sunset.

If you could smell, taste, hear, or see any of those things, then you were stimulating your sensory memories. We do this naturally when we daydream, when we are bored, or when we are remembering a situation that occurred, both pleasant and unpleasant. Often people review the unpleasant situations that have been left unfinished or unresolved. They mull them over and think about what could have been done differently or better, or finally come up with that snappy comeback that they wished they had used. Disoriented elderly do this as well, often with a greater sense of urgency because they are striving to find peace before they die.

The principle is important to remember when disoriented elderly say that they see or hear someone or something that is not really there. They have stimulated the visual or auditory memory as part of the scene that they are replaying. Because they have let go of present-day reality, the past has become more vibrant, and there is a need to resolve, retreat, relive, or relieve; the disoriented older person calls forth people or things from the past to fulfill the pressing need in the moment.

People Live on Several Levels of Awareness, Often at the Same Time

This interesting phenomenon occurs in everyday life usually without awareness of it. Levels of awareness range from unconsciousness to hyper-awareness—the half-asleep dozing on a warm sunny beach in the summer versus walking down a dark, unfamiliar street in a strange city. Often when we are in a less aware state of consciousness (sleeping or half asleep), a part of us remains alert for the unexpected or for potential danger. People who have had children know what it is like to wake up suddenly out of a deep sleep at the first cry of the baby. This duality of awareness is useful. For very old disoriented people, this ability to be aware on at least two levels at the same time comes in handy when they are using their "mind's eye" to see someone from the past. They "see" the wished-for person, yet on some unconscious level know that the person is not there. Naomi Feil told me the story of an old woman in a nursing facility who pointed to an empty door and said, "Oh look, there's my mother. I have to go to her." The nurse said to her, "Mrs. Smith, you are 89 years old. Your mother passed on a while ago." The old woman responded, "Well, I know that and you know that, but my mother doesn't know that and that's why I have to go to her!"

For caregivers, it is important to trust that the disoriented person knows the "truth" of reality on some level. Never lie or pretend that you see what is not there. Never play along with the "fantasy" of the disoriented person. She knows what is real. She knows on a preconscious level whether you are pretending or lying. Do not break down the trust in the relationship.

When Present Reality Becomes Painful, Some Elderly People Survive by Retreating and Stimulating Memories of the Past

This is one of the coping strategies that everyone uses to some extent at difficult moments in life. When the situation becomes too painful or difficult, people withdraw. Some people use this coping mechanism more frequently than others. Some are able to repress totally the current reality and ignore it completely. This often is seen at traumatic accident scenes or when one cannot escape from an uncomfortable situation (e.g., a very long, boring meeting). As mentioned previously, very old people resolve, retreat, relive, or relieve. Retreating from a reality in which one feels isolated, misunderstood, unappreciated, and put upon is normal and understandable. For very old disoriented people, it can be seen as a healthy response that helps them in fulfilling the final life task.

Feelings Experienced in the Present Can Trigger Memories of Having Felt Similarly in the Past

Everyone has experienced this principle at various times in life. For example, my daughter yells at me for not allowing her to stay out late, and, in response, I blow up and yell at her. Normally such an adolescent flare-up would not annoy me so much, but this situation is similar to three other events that happened in the past month when I did not express my anger and controlled it. The anger from the three earlier events is triggered and joins into an angry outburst. Emotionally tinged memories are powerful, especially when the feelings have been repressed or ignored.

Painful Feelings that Are Expressed, Acknowledged, and Validated by a Trusted Listener Will Diminish; Painful Feelings that Are Ignored or Suppressed Will Gain in Strength

Anger, sadness, fear, frustration, and hurt are painful emotions, or are sometimes called *negative feelings.* Some people can express these feelings when they come up; some people think that they should not express negative feelings or have concern that by expressing these feelings things will get worse. "If I start crying, then I'll never stop"; "If I get angry, then I might hurt someone"; "It doesn't make the pain go away if I complain about it." These are commonly heard concerns that reflect an underlying fear of losing control. Expressing feelings can feel like letting go or like opening a dam after a heavy rain. That is not a bad metaphor for what happens when feelings are held back. The feelings are dammed up. If they do not get released, then they will overflow the banks. Water that is left standing in a pool for a long time without movement becomes brackish, dark, and smelly. Once the water is allowed to flow, it takes awhile before it will flow clean and before the built-up pressure is released enough to allow for gentle movement instead of a gush.

Mrs. Samdan was in a Japanese concentration camp in her native Indonesia. She survived and lived a relatively normal life, but now in a nursing facility, she weeps daily, complains of pains throughout her body (doctors have found no physical cause for the pains), and talks on and on about her internment to anyone who will listen. She needs to express her pain on a daily basis, and that may continue until she dies. The intensity of the expression will lessen as she is given opportunity to express. If those around her do not listen or try to stop her, then the feelings will remain under pressure and painful.

The simple act of listening to someone express painful feelings is powerful. Listening acutely and with caring is sometimes more difficult than it seems. Listening with empathy, actually sharing the feelings that are being expressed by the other, is most effective. This is the key element of Validation.

Listening with Empathy Builds Trust, Reduces Anxiety, and Restores Dignity

When faced with moving our family from one country to another, I experienced a series of panic attacks; I felt overwhelmed with too much to do and too much responsibility. I tried talking about my irrational fears to some people, who began to offer me advice on how to make it work better. Some explained to me why my fears were irrational, and others quickly changed the subject to something else. It was pointless to express my feelings to someone who did not want to hear them. I felt worse when not taken seriously or when my feelings were avoided. When I did speak with someone who listened to me and accepted my feelings, I was able to "get it off my chest" and eventually felt better. The anxiety went away; I felt validated.

Valid means "well grounded or justifiable; being at once relevant and meaningful"; *validate* means "to support or corroborate on a sound or authoritative basis" (*Webster's Dictionary*). The Validation method is based on supporting the emotional reality of other people—finding the relevance and meaning of the emotions.

WHAT DO THE BEHAVIORS OF DISORIENTED VERY OLD PEOPLE MEAN?

If one accepts the premise that there is a reason for all behavior, then it is logical to accept that the reason for behavior has something to do with needs and desires. Very old disoriented people have needs and desires that are not so different from those of oriented and younger people. Using Maslow's classic hierarchy of needs (Atkinson & Atkinson) as a guideline, here are some ideas of what could be the relevance of your disoriented relative's behavior.

Everyone has basic physiological needs for food, drink, and shelter. Also included in this basic level are the needs for sexual stimulation and sensory stimulation. Although many people find it embarrassing or hard to believe, sexual needs do not stop when you hit 65 years of age. Sexual feelings continue on some level until death. The intensity of the need is individual: Some elderly feel a great deal of sexual need, and some less so, which is not so different from younger people. No one does well in isolation or in situations in which there is sensory deprivation. This is considered a form of torture, actually. Very old people often experience a significant deterioration of the sensory systems: Hearing diminishes (especially the higher tones); vision becomes reduced; the sense of taste changes as a result of decreased sensitivity in the receptors, and various medications (frequently given to very old people) affect the sense of taste in that foods taste metallic or sour; the sense of touch can be affected by a reduction in sensitivity in the fingertips or by poor circulation; sense of balance and kinesthetic awareness of one's place in space are affected by medications (sedatives or psychotropic drugs) or by damage to particular areas of the brain through small strokes or simple deterioration that comes with age; the sense of smell is probably the least affected by the aging process, although this, too, deteriorates to some degree in old age. Less information is available from the environment. These reductions in sensory input create a sensory isolation. The here-and-now reality becomes blurred, dim, tasteless, dull, and insecure.

The need to feel safe and secure does not change as we grow older; in fact, it sometimes heightens. The need to be nurtured grows as one feels more vulnerable. This is not the same as the need to be mothered, which often is confused with nurturing. One can nurture without mothering. Nurturing is helping the other grow; in this context, it has to do with growing more secure and feeling loved. Older people who have diminished sensory input often feel more out of touch with the environment and so less safe and secure. Elderly who are not stable when they walk are sometimes "fixed" to their chairs (i.e., physically restrained) to keep them from walking. Although this may seem to offer security, most elderly people experience physical restraints as frightening and less safe, as imprisonment rather than security.

Many older people who express themselves in bizarre ways (not readily understandable), who yell or move around a lot, are given medications to calm them. Chemical restraints (sedatives or psychotropic drugs) forcibly repress emotions and the person's ability to express them. It can feel like a hijacking of one's ability to communicate. It creates frustration and anger, then depression and withdrawal. This is a far cry from safe and secure. Most often it is the caregivers who feel insecure with the disoriented person's expression of feelings. It is our fears that must be quelled and our anxiety and insecurity that need to be addressed.

Everyone can relate to the need to be loved and to be affiliated with other people; "no man is an island." Deep unhappiness comes from isolation and a dearth of love. Very old people are left bereft when they have lost many of their loved ones, many of their friends, their social circles, and their sources for love and association. Making new friends does not take the place of having old friends. Friendship is different from love that flows from bonds that are made early in one's personal history. There is no replacement for those relationships. Affiliation, or the feeling that one gets when part of a larger group, is related to work situations, professional associations, and social groups, such as being part of a neighborhood or more formalized in societies or clubs. Humans are social animals who need to belong to a larger whole to see themselves as worthwhile individuals—an interesting paradox. When one is taken out of the whole, the feeling of being ostracized, shut out, or left by the wayside often diminishes a person's feelings of worth. Many older people lose their affiliations with familiar groups and, with that, a part of their self-worth.

Recognition and respect from others contributes to feeling worthwhile. Self-worth is derived partially from how one is treated by others. For some people, this is crucial, whereas for others, it is less important. Recognition and respect come from personal relationships as well as from the community. Recognition from a community often is in the form of status. When one has status, others listen to what is said. One is spoken to in a respectful form and voice tone; one's achievements are noted. A person who has reached very old age has a lifetime of achievements and experience. The need for recognition, respect, and status may not change, but society certainly changes the way that it values older people. Disoriented very old people lose even more status when they do not conform to social rules, but their need to be appreciated for who they are and what they have done in their life remains. Too many disoriented elderly are treated as though they are children, addressing them with their first names or with pet names, such as "honey" or "sweetie." Too many people use a parental or condescending voice tone. Too many people think that just because a person forgets or does not know where she is, the need for respect and recognition is lost. It is in fact more crucial in this last stage of life than perhaps at any other stage.

Understanding the world and exploring it is a need that drives some people in their professions or hobbies. The desire to travel to foreign countries, to try bungee jumping, or to discover the genome is not felt by everyone. A slightly less intense version of this, felt universally, is the need to have a clear understanding of the immediate environment—to know how it works and the relationships that are involved; to be familiar with the patterns, values, and rhythms. Think of a time when you started a new job in a new company. One first has to learn the physical layout: where the bathrooms are, your work area, the coffee pot, and so forth. Then one explores the people and their relationships: who your colleagues are, the boss; who is friendly, who is not. As you gather information, you begin to feel comfortable (hopefully). Very old disoriented people also experience this need to make sense of their environment and the people around them. If the disoriented person is at home, then it is easy to think, "Oh, my mother is in a familiar place; she won't have this problem," but, actually, if the person is reliving experiences from another time or retreating to a time and place where she felt useful, or is relieving the pain of being old and useless or resolving an unfinished issue from long ago, then the here and now does not fit with what is going on in her mind's eye. The differences between the environment and the personal reality create dissonance. If the person is in a facility, then often the dissonance is greater. There is the added factor of strangers in the environment, strangers being people who do not fit into the personal reality. Very old people strive to make sense of a strange and sometimes unbearable reality and to find a place that feels comfortable, where relationships and people are familiar.

Symmetry, order, and beauty create an aesthetic aspect to life. Some people feel this need more than others. Artists and designers fulfill this need as part of their daily lives. Most people incorporate some aesthetics into their life by creating a lovely home environment, going to museums or the theater, listening to music, lighting candles, and so forth. Aesthetics give harmony and balance. Very old people also seek harmony and balance, but fulfilling this need becomes more complicated because eyesight, hearing, mobility, and memory fail. How does one find harmony amidst the cacophony of an institutional life? How does one find balance when one cannot stand up? How does one incorporate beauty into a life that is concerned primarily with deficits? One does not. Disoriented old-old retreat from the ugliness or dissonance and instead relive moments of harmony from the past. It also is possible for some disoriented elderly simply to apply the picture in their mind's eye to reality, like putting on rose-colored glasses. They see what they want to see and hear what they want to hear. The caregiver becomes the daughter whose very presence gives pleasure and a sense of well-being. Napkins become the canvas and orange juice the paint when the desire to be creative needs to be expressed.

Self-actualization is the need at the top of Maslow's pyramid, something that many people strive to achieve but that few actually accomplish. The desire to become a better person, to reach maximum potential, drives many to self-help books, therapy, adult education courses, meditation, and so many other development-oriented activities. The need to develop often declines as people grow older. They often become more accommodating to what is and more resistant to change. In old age, the need seems to shift from forward thinking to reflection on the past. Summing up what was and coming to terms with the choices that one has made can be seen as a variation on the self-actualization theme. This desire to find peace with oneself becomes a driving force for many very old people, particularly when they are disoriented. Feil called this need *resolution*. Many disoriented old-old strive on a preconscious level to resolve unfinished issues before they die. It is a process that continues until the end.

RESOLUTION: THE TASKS OF LIFE'S FINAL PHASE

In Validation theory, Feil describes the final life stage: resolution. In this stage of life, people struggle to resolve unfinished "business" so that they can die in peace. It is a process, not an end point. The opposite of resolving is moving deeper and deeper inward, withdrawing from reality and the surroundings. Feil describes four phases of this process: malorientation, time confusion, repetitive motion, and finally, vegetation. Disoriented very old people do not necessarily go through all four phases. It is not always progressive. In fact, in many cases, people have gone from repetitive motion to time confusion or from time confusion to malorientation, but in no case that I know of has a person become completely oriented. The four phases describe a process of retreating from the here and now, from the people around them, from what is going on, and from the environment. It is a survival mechanism that is totally connected to a deep need to resolve, retreat, relive, and relieve. There is little in reality that satisfies these needs. In fact, there is much in reality that drives disoriented very old people to withdraw further.

Malorientation

The first phase of resolution is malorientation. People who are in this phase are oriented to reality, meaning that they usually know where they are, who they are, who you are, what time it is, and so forth, but they have an aspect of their personality that is dysfunctional. They are aware of their inability to cope with their aging process on some level, but they cannot admit it. They cling to what they have, fearful of losing more. The normally occurring changes that happen as people age become unacceptable infringements on a person's identity, honor, and self-worth. For instance, I was always called "eagle-eye Rubin" because I could see clearly, very far. Now, at age 48, I have difficulty reading a map in the car. I can accept that my eyesight has deteriorated and that I am no longer "eagle-eye Rubin," or I can deny that loss because it is too painful to give up that important part of my identity. I can blame the maps or the signs for being written unclearly or too small. If remembering things is an important part of who I am—"I remember everything"—then forgetting things becomes a sign not only of aging but also of a loss of identity. If I cannot handle that, then I need to deny it, repress it, or blame something or someone else. This is what underlies malorientation. Those who are in malorientation use denial, repression, blame, and sometimes even hopelessness to a dysfunctional extreme. The following are examples of people in malorientation.

> Mrs. White (age: 87) lives alone not too far from her daughter, Nancy. Since Mrs. White's husband died 2 years ago, she has begun complaining that she has trouble breathing, particularly in the middle of the night. Often she calls Nancy at 2:00 or 3:00 A.M. in panic, demanding that she come over right away. When the daughter comes over a half hour later, Mrs. White answers the door and complains angrily that Nancy has awakened her. Mrs. White also gets very angry when Nancy goes away on business trips. Mrs. White calls her daughter when Nancy is away to say that she is dying and if Nancy does not come home right away, she'll be dead.

✻

> Mr. Johnson (age: 89) lives with his son and daughter-in-law and their two children. Sometimes he goes to his old office building,

where he used to work as a lawyer, dressed in a suit and carrying an old briefcase. When the office staff reminds him that he is long retired, he responds, "Well, I know that. I'm just checking up on you." He constantly criticizes his 13-year-old granddaughter, warning her that her choice of clothes will get her into trouble. When his son asks him to respect the children's privacy, Mr. Johnson launches into a tirade of abusive warnings. His daughter-in-law eases the tension, but the situation is worsening.

❁

Mrs. Gold (age: 85) lives with her daughter, Anne, who is divorced and has a teenage son. Anne is having difficulty with her mother because she goes to the neighbors complaining that they have put garbage in her garden. Some of the neighbors have become very angry and called the police. Mrs. Gold argues with the police and shows them the backyard, which is clean, saying that the neighbors took all of the garbage away when they called the police. She claims that they are trying to make her crazy and have her put away. Anne has been called repeatedly at work and told she needs to do something.

Time Confusion

The second phase of resolution is time confusion. In this phase, the person is no longer oriented to time, place, or person. This means that the person may not know where she is, who you are, or which day it is. People who are in time confusion are still able to talk and communicate verbally but have let go of common reality in exchange for a "personal reality." They are poetic and often very creative in expressing themselves and their needs. They no longer abide by social conventions or rules when those get in the way of expression. Social conventions guide when to eat, how to eat, how to dress, how to greet people, what to say, and what is acceptable behavior and what is not acceptable. Forsaking social rules often is what disturbs others because these rules are so important to society.

For instance, if an older woman wants to "go home to her parents" because she feels lost and alone, she may put on her hat and coat and then walk up and down the halls inside; in her mind, she turns those halls into the streets of her youth. A woman looks out the window on the second floor of a locked dementia unit and says, "Oh look. What a pretty porch. You could sit out on that porch and rock." She is remembering the porch of a house from earlier in her life and the feeling of sitting in the sun; rocking is much more pleasant than sitting in a depressing, white-walled locked unit across from drooling, disoriented neighbors. The following are examples of people in time confusion.

Mrs. Banner (age: 86) has always been a very friendly woman. She lives with her daughter and goes out every day and greets everyone she meets as though they were her old friends from her youth. She often gets lost and cannot find her way back home, not even knowing what city she is in. She thinks that she lives in New Jersey, where she was a girl. She flirts in a girlish way with all of the men who come to the house and with the policeman who has had to bring her home several times. She tells the same old stories about all of the boyfriends she has.

❋

Mrs. MacNamara (age: 91) lives with her husband (age: 93), who has been caring for her since she became "confused" approximately 4 years ago. She sometimes does not recognize him and thinks that he is a burglar. She screams and demands that he get out of the house and leave her alone. Sometimes she hits him. She had always been a highly controlled and controlling woman, but now she cannot control herself. She lashes out at everyone, driving them away. Even the nurses who come every day to help her get dressed in the morning are verbally attacked.

❋

Mr. Walker (age: 85) lives alone in the same small town as his four children, who take turns caring for him every day. He responds to all women by flirting with them and making sexual comments about their appearance. Even his daughter gets patted on the bottom sometimes, when he does not recognize her as his daughter. Mr. Walker finds sexual references in everything and is very vocal about it. Sometimes he masturbates when other people are present. His children are embarrassed; they do not want to take him out of the house and do not know what to do.

Repetitive Motion

Repetitive motion is the third phase of resolution. People in repetitive motion have stopped communicating primarily with words. They express themselves through movements or sounds. Their need to express themselves is as strong as yours or mine, but they have lost the capacity or motivation to interact with "reality," with people, and with the environment. People in repetitive motion have withdrawn into themselves even further than those in time confusion. This means that they do not often take note of what or who is around them. They are caught up in their own world, which is an expression of their needs. The repetitive movements and sounds are in fact a part of that expression of feelings —the need to be useful (working) or to belong. Movements of the mouth can create feelings; the use of new word combinations, which may sound like gibberish to us, actually is a unique way of saying what needs to be said. The following are examples of people in repetitive motion.

Mrs. Xavier (age: 92) walks through the halls of the nursing facility where she has lived for the past year. Her daughter could not care for her at home when Mrs. Xavier withdrew from all contact with others and became totally incontinent and dependent on her daughter for washing, dressing, and eating. Mrs. Xavier lumbers on her still-strong legs, stopping occasionally to pick up a tissue, a pen, a fork, or any other item that she passes on her way. She does not look up when people greet her and speaks only when directly confronted with a simple question, such as, "Do you want a cup of coffee?" Her eyes are usually cast downward, and she seems to be in "another world." To understand her personal reality, it is important to know that Mrs. Xavier lived in a town that was bombed during World War II and had to care for her two children alone because her husband had been killed in action.

Each day was filled with fear and the desperate search for food and clothing.

Mr. Peters (age: 88) is at home being cared for by his daughter-in-law. He is totally dependent on her and the visiting nurse who helps each day with getting him washed and dressed. Once he is in his big chair in the living room, he sits the entire day pounding on the table in front of him or rubbing his hand back and forth across the table top. Sometimes he will take an object and roll it around in his hand for a long time. Mr. Peters does not speak much, but sometimes one can hear words such as, "Good," or, "That's right." For those who know that Mr. Peters had his own carpentry business and for 60 years created beautiful hand-made furniture, his behavior begins to make sense.

Mrs. Clark (age: 84) is kept tied in her wheelchair because she keeps wanting to get up and walk. The nursing staff in the facility where she lives worries that she will fall and break a hip if she walks around. Mrs. Clark spends her day folding her dress, napkins, the tablecloth, or any other soft, flat thing that she can reach. Softly she hums parts of old children's songs and sometimes says things that no one can understand in a voice tone that sounds like a mother talking to small children. At 3:00 P.M. each afternoon (when school is out), she becomes restless and calls out, "Help." Her children do not come to visit her often because they do not know what to do and do not have the feeling that it helps her at all. She does not recognize them or talk with them. What they do not realize is that Mrs. Clark was at her happiest when she was a young mother of three small children, busy taking care of them, and in fact had built her life around their well-being and happiness.

Vegetation

The final phase of resolution is vegetation. This is a complete withdrawal from reality. People in vegetation lie or sit without moving, without speaking, and without connection to what is around them. They are fully dependent on others for care. We do not understand what is going on inside the minds of people who are in vegetation, because they no longer communicate. It is very difficult to make contact with these people, and that is why one of the goals of Validation is to prevent vegetation. Reactions are minimal—the blink of an eye, a moment of real eye contact, perhaps the movement of fingers or feet, but that is all. It is a pre-death state of being, but one that can last for years.

There are many different reasons for why people decline or withdraw into deeper stages of disorientation. Sometimes there is a physical reason for the decline: a stroke that leaves lasting damage to the brain, paralysis, or the loss of speech; the loss of sensory information because eyesight, hearing, touch, taste, and smell have diminished. If information does not enter the system, then it is more difficult to orient oneself. An example of this is when you wake up sleepy in a strange bed in a strange place. There often is a moment of confusion until the sensory system wakes up and gives enough information to orient yourself. Lack of sensory input is isolating and sometimes scary. For example, a man does not put in his hearing aid because it is uncomfortable and so misses out on conversation and feels cut off from family. Instead of spending the energy to try to communicate (it takes a lot of energy), he simply follows his own thoughts and stops communicating with those around him.

There are psychological losses that can be too overwhelming. The death of a spouse, the loss of a child, and moving to other living quarters are three major life changes that often are a significant trigger for withdrawal. As a mother, I cannot imagine a pain worse than losing my child. Having seen relatives handle the loss of their 12-year-old son, I became more aware of the enormous psychological flexibility and strength that it takes to go through such a crisis and come out functioning and able to go on. When some women lose a husband on whom they have based their lives, the foundation crumbles. Some men have been dependent on their wives for everything, and when she goes, they are left unable to care for themselves and become despondent. It takes psychological strength and flexibility to handle this crisis. Some people are very connected to the place where they live. They have lived their entire adult life there, and often significant memories are attached to that place. A house also could be a sign of status or a symbol of their security. Losing one's home can be devastating. It often is the move from home that triggers disorientation, especially when the individual is moved to an institution. Institutional living can create increased disorientation simply because of what it is not: not "home," not safe, not familiar, not private, and often not the choice of the individual who is moved there. It takes enormous resources and skills to handle these types of psychological losses, and often people reach old age unable to cope with them.

Social losses are added to this growing pile of losses that come with aging. Social losses have to do with our role in society—the place that we have had and the place that we now occupy. Depending on the situation, this societal role can be significant and have great value to the extent that one's identity is bonded to that role. Many people experience a loss of importance when they retire. Without work, they are worthless. For some, the loss of a social network because of the death of friends becomes too much to handle, and they are isolated.

CONCLUSION

Everyone has ways of coping with difficulties that life brings. Some coping mechanisms work better than others in differing circumstances. If one has a broad palate of ways of coping, then one can better adapt as one gets older.

Within an institution, older people often are treated in ways that increase disorientation rather than motivate them to stay in the "here and now" or to communicate with those around them. Living in communal bedrooms (six-bed rooms still exist) is confusing and depersonalizing. Use of sedatives to help people sleep or to keep them quiet makes for a forced withdrawal into an inner world. Psychotropic drugs (antipsychotic medication) often are given when older people say that they see something or hear something that staff members do not see or hear or when elderly people behave in ways that staff does not appreciate. These drugs repress the identity and create disorientation. Out of fear that the older person will fall and hurt herself, the staff often restrains those who constantly walk. Restraints can be in the form of padded bands around a chair or placement in a chair that has a tray. For a person who needs to move, these restraints are torture. For a person who needs to express herself, sedatives or other repressing medications can feel like drowning. Is it any wonder that a person withdraws inward? Reality is too painful. It gives nothing that she needs. There is nothing to gain by remaining in a torturous circumstance, and that often is why people decline further into disorientation and move into deeper phases of resolution.

Part II

How to Communicate
with Your Disoriented Relative

Validation is a method for communicating with disoriented very old people. The theory on which this method is based provides the starting point. If you accept the principles discussed in Part I and recognize the needs that are expressed by disoriented elderly people, then you have a sturdy base for using Validation. The base is the attitude with which one approaches other people. In Validation, a person uses empathy to enter the personal world of a disoriented person. Empathy is the ability to put your own feelings aside and to take on the feelings of another to share her feelings for awhile. It is not acting; it is not faking, pretending, or projecting. This may sound simple, but in fact it can be the most difficult aspect of using Validation. The following is a summary of how to validate:

- Center

- Observe

- Find the appropriate distance

- Find empathy

- Use appropriate verbal and nonverbal techniques

- End the conversation on a positive note

CENTER

Each time you want to validate, you need to *center*. This means clearing yourself of all of the inner "noise," putting aside your own feelings, quieting the thoughts that are running through your head, and finding your inner strength and resourcefulness. If you meditate, do yoga, or do some form of martial arts, then these words are familiar to you. You may already be trained in centering, and that is an extremely important tool that you will need to use often. If this is new to you, then please spend time learning to center. Centering is what you do when you do not know what to do. Centering is the way to handle shocking, scary events. Centering is the first step toward empathy. There are many exercises that you can use to practice. Here is an example:

1. Imagine your feet firmly planted and connected to the earth.

2. Create an imaginary connection between the top of your head and the universe, perhaps visualize a trail of stars or a rainbow.

3. Create a connection between your coccyx (tail bone) and the earth, anchoring yourself to the earth.

4. Visualize your spine as a strand of pearls hanging from the topmost pearl, and allow the pearls to align themselves one under the other. As you align your spine, you will feel the strength and centeredness. You can always test this by imag-

ining one pearl out of alignment and feel the difference in your body. Realign those pearls to regain the center and the strength.

If the words that are used in this exercise do not work for you, that does not matter. Find your own way. It does not matter how you get there. Different centering exercises are listed in Appendix 3.

OBSERVE

Once you are centered, you need to observe your disoriented relative carefully. You can do this from a distance. Observe the following:

- The hair: Is it combed or messy?
- The eyes: Are they wide open, expressive of a particular emotion or of tension?
- The forehead: Are the eyebrows pointing up or down?
- The nose: Is it thinned, or are the nostrils flared?
- The lips: Are they pursed, bitten, in a smile?
- The jaw: Is it tensed or relaxed?
- The mouth: Which emotion is being reflected by the shape of the mouth?
- The shoulders: Are they pulled up, down, forward, backward, slumped?
- The chest: How is the person breathing: fast, slow, high in the chest, or low in the belly?
- The body position: Does the posture reflect an emotion or state of being?
- The arms and hands: Are they tense or relaxed; is there movement?

- The legs and feet: Are they tense or relaxed, open or closed, pulled in or spread out?

- Movements in space: Are they direct or indirect, gracious or stiff?

The key is to identify a state of being. The more information that you can glean by simply observing, the easier it will be to make your initial approach. As you approach the person, centered and observing, try to match her; that is, take on some of the physical characteristics yourself. Perhaps you can breathe in the same rhythm, wrinkle your brow in the same way, or reflect the emotion that you sense is coming from the other person. Learning to recognize and reflect emotions is difficult for some people, but it is the next crucial step in communicating.

Recognizing feelings from nonverbal clues can be difficult if you are not used to it. Here's an exercise. The following pictures of people's faces reflect different emotions. Try to identify the emotion, and specifically notice the facial features.

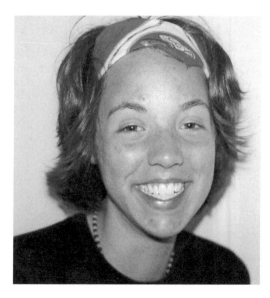

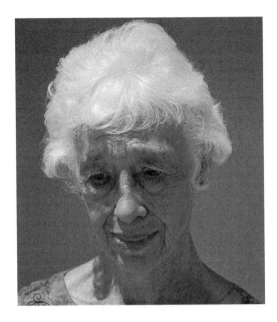

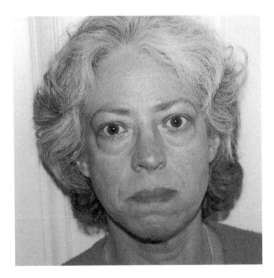

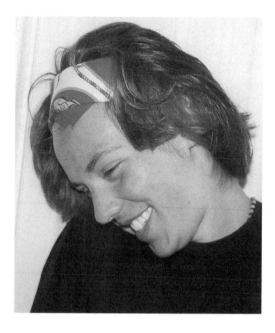

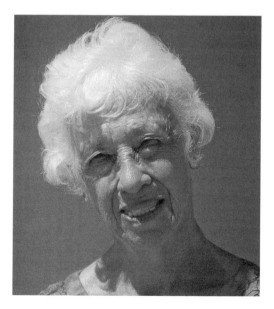

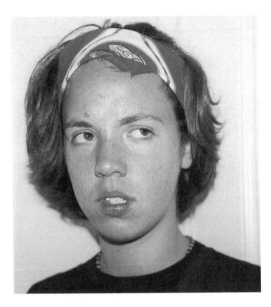

FIND THE APPROPRIATE DISTANCE

A person in malorientation usually needs normal social distance until there is trust and an intimate relationship. Please note that even if you are the partner, son, or sister of this person, this does not automatically allow you physical closeness. It is extremely important for you to center and put your needs aside so that you can be aware of the needs of the other. A person who is in time confusion (phase 2, as described in Part I) generally will need more closeness. Because she has let go of social controls and rules, a woman who is in phase 2 more easily accepts nearness. Because she has withdrawn inward into her own world, you need to get close to make contact. Experience shows that the energy field that surrounds a person who is in time confusion is approximately 8 inches, but because each person is individual and has individual needs, one has to "feel the way in" to making contact. People who are in repetitive motion (phase 3) have withdrawn even further, and to make contact, one must get even closer. Touching the person often is needed simply to be acknowledged as being present. Those who are in vegetation (phase 4) require the most closeness. They have pulled their energy field totally inward. This often is experienced as "not being there." Touch is crucial for making contact.

FIND EMPATHY

It is at this stage of making contact with the person whom you want to validate that you need to develop empathy. Empathy is more than being interested in the other person. Empathy is more than feeling sympathy for the other person. Empathy is actually feeling the emotions that the other person is feeling in the moment. You have centered and cleared your own thoughts and feelings. You have observed which emotions are going on in the other person. As you move toward the other, feeling your way into an appropriate position, you also need to feel your way into the emotion. For some, this is easy; for others, it is very difficult. This is not play-acting. This is not labeling someone by saying, "she is angry" or "he is sad." Many people feel empathy once they have adjusted their facial expression to match the other person. Finding empathy is a process: observation, incorporation, reverberation, and then afterwards, detachment. The actual moment of feeling emotion arises when one incorporates the other person. *Reverberation* is the expression of that feeling through your own facial expression, body position, voice tone, and energy. *Detachment* is letting go of the other person's emotions, clearing yourself by centering, and allowing your own feelings to come back.

USE APPROPRIATE VERBAL AND NONVERBAL TECHNIQUES

The communication techniques that are used in Validation come from a number of sources and are used in various forms of therapy. Having a broad range of communication techniques gives you more possibilities for contact. The following are techniques that are most useful for each phase of resolution. Practice two or three of them that are most comfortable for you and that seem to work best with your relative.

Techniques that Work Best with People Who Are in Malorientation

Use open questions. Questions that cannot be answered "yes" or "no" usually begin with "who," "what," "where," "when," or "how." Avoid using "why" questions.

Open questions explore what is important in the moment. They stimulate conversation. Normal social phrases, such as, "How are you?" and "What's going on?" are good ways to begin. Note that turning statements into questions with a raised voice tone does not count as an open question (e.g., "You seem upset, huh?").

Using closed questions is okay but limiting. A closed question can be answered with "yes" or "no" (e.g., "Are you alright?"). Too many closed questions can feel like an interview rather than a conversation and will stimulate feelings of suspicion: "Why are you asking me all these questions? What do you want from me?" It is normal and fine to ask closed questions once in awhile, but try to follow the closed question with an open question: "Are you alright?" "What's going on?" "Where does it hurt?"

The question "why" is missing from the list for a very good reason. Asking why a person feels or thinks a particular way does not help the person express him- or herself. It is a request for an explanation for our benefit; it serves our need to understand. Most often, the person does not know why she thinks or feels a certain way. The question "why" asks for cognitive ability and insight, capacities that often are missing in malorientation and certainly missing in disorientation. Asking "why" can be confronting and often creates irritation, anger, or frustration. It does not help stimulate a trusting relationship and intimate communication. The following is an example:

Vicki: Good morning, Mrs. C. How are you today?

Mrs. C: Terrible. (*frowning and tense*)

Vicki: What happened?

Mrs. C: All my things were stolen.

Vicki: What are you missing?

Mrs. C: My jewelry.

Vicki: Do you know who took it?

Mrs. C: That nurse, the one with the dark hair.

Rephrase what the person has just said, using her key words (i.e., the words that are emphasized by voice tone), the words that carry some emotional weight. Rephrasing is not just repeating what was just said to fill a silent gap. Rephrasing must be done with empathy and concentration; otherwise, it can feel as though one is being mimicked. The point of rephrasing is to show the other person that you really understand on a deep level what she is saying. When one has correctly rephrased, the other person feels understood and accepted, often exclaiming, "Exactly!"

Mrs. C: She always comes into *my* room and takes *my* things.

Vicki: She takes *your* things from *your* room?

Mrs. C: You bet!

Ask the extreme, meaning, find out the boundaries of what is going on. Use words such as "always" and "never," or ask how often or how much.

Vicki: How often does she do that?

Mrs. C: Every day.

Vicki: Does she take everything or one thing at a time?

Explore the opposite. Find out what would happen if the opposite were true.

Vicki: Is there a time when she doesn't come into your room and take things?

Mrs. C: Now that you mention it, when you're around she doesn't do it.

Reminiscing about the past is easy and pleasurable to do with your relative when she is in the mood for that. There are many ways to do this. You can go through or create photo albums, help her write an autobiography, or simply ask about common events from the past. "Do you remember when . . . ?" You can also explore more by asking questions such as, "What was the most important moment in your life?" "What was the happiest moment?" "What was the most difficult moment?"

Finding a familiar coping mechanism can help your relative deal with a current problem. Often, problems repeat in our life, and strategies that helped us in the past can be useful in the present. For instance,

Mrs. C: I can't sleep. That racket from the neighbors keeps me up all night long.

Vicki: Did that ever happen before?

Mrs. C: When we lived in that old apartment, the cheap one with walls thin as paper; we could hear everything.

Vicki: What did you do then?

Mrs. C: Well, your dad never minded the noise, but I would use ear plugs sometimes. You know you can roll little pieces of toilet tissue and make really good ear plugs.

Vicki: Could you make those ear plugs now? Do you think they might help?

Mrs. C: I had forgotten about that. Bring me a piece of toilet tissue, and I'll show you how I did it.

There is one last technique that can be used, the *preferred sense.* This technique is more complicated to explain and more subtle in use. It comes from neurolinguistic programming, which is a practical model for human communication and change that was developed by two Californians in the mid-1970s. It begins with the awareness that most people have a preferred sense (sight, sound, smell, taste, or touch) that comes into play more frequently or is the first filter of information. We "see" what the other person means or "hear" what the other is saying, or the information

Sensory words

Visual	Auditory	Kinesthetic	Nonsensory
See, view	Loud/soft	Feel	Think, seem
Dark/light	Ringing	Warm/cold	Wonder
Cloudy, misty	Ask, speak, say,	Soft/hard	Find
Clear, bright	hear	Pressure	Want
Blind	Sing, tone, hum	Touch	Good/bad
Red, blue, green,	Noise	Sensitive	Nice, fun
etc.	Snore	Excited, tense	Unpleasant
Glittering	Banging,	Smooth/rough	
Stare	scratch	Dry/wet, damp	
	Drumming		
	Quiet		

"hits" you in a hard way. When you speak to another person using her preferred sense, the information or communication makes a better connection. For example, if you know that someone is a visual person you can say, "What does it look like to you?" You are more likely to get a response when you "speak the same language" than if you "need to be translated." Using the preferred sense is a way of building trust more quickly and making communication easier.

The easiest way to identify someone's preferred sense is to listen to the word choices that the person makes. Does he or she use visual words often? Try to listen for the sensory words. The table above has some suggestions to help you.

Once you have identified the preferred sense, use it when you explore the other person's situation.

Mrs. C: You know, that neighbor of mine is keeping me up all night with her *racket*. I haven't slept in days.

Vicki: What does it *sound* like?

Mrs. C: Well, first there's a loud crash, like she's pushing furniture. She doesn't walk, she stomps to the bathroom, and then there's the sound of water running all the time and flushing. That woman must pee all night long.

Summary of Techniques for People who Communicate Verbally

Use open questions: who, what, where, when, or how.

Rephrase what the person has said; use key words.

Ask about the extreme.

Reminisce about the past.

Find a familiar coping mechanism.

Use the preferred sense.

Techniques that Work Best with People Who Are in Time Confusion and Repetitive Motion

If a disoriented person communicates verbally, then you can use all of the previously described techniques. When using questioning techniques with people who have limited verbal ability, it is important to shift from primarily asking open questions, which are difficult to answer if one has aphasia, for instance, or other damage to the speech centers of the brain. In this case, it is better to *ask closed questions*—questions that can be answered with "yes" or "no." Use words that are easy for the person to grasp or relate to because of their personal history (e.g., work-related terms). It is also good to *offer two possible answers as choices.* For instance,

Mrs. C: (*looking sad, eyes cast down, body slumped a bit forward in her chair, rubbing her hand on the table surface in a slow, brushing movement*)

Vicki: Mrs. C, you're looking sad. Is it that you miss being at home or miss working?

I choose these two "needs" because I know Mrs. C's history and that being at home with her children and being active were two very important issues for her throughout her life.

If a person communicates minimally with words, then concentrate on the following nonverbal techniques.

Mirroring is reflecting the same posture, physical movements, facial expression, voice tone, and even breathing as the other person. Just one element can be mirrored or all of them. Mirroring in Validation is not the same as mimicking. Mimicking is simply copying for the sake of copying. Mirroring has the intention of developing empathy and communicating in a nonverbal manner. Often, mirroring a repetitive motion can provide a better understanding of the meaning behind the behavior. It is truly moving into the inner world of the other person.

Genuine, deep eye contact is the beginning to every deep or intimate relationship. It will connect you. Getting on eye level with the other person, getting physically close, and then observing the person's face and eyes very carefully is an invitation for eye contact.

Use *touch* to make contact with a person who is withdrawn deeply into her own world. A gentle touch on the arm or shoulder is a way of connecting. Always remember first to make sure that the person knows that you are there. Say, "Hello," or some other greeting, and then move in close. Try to get eye contact and gently start to touch with the goal of making contact and building a relationship. Another type of touching is *anchored touch.* This is based on the concept of *anchoring,* which is the connection between an emotional state and a physical sensation—in this case, the connection between an emotion and a touch. Feil discovered that most older people react to a certain type of touch on the cheek by remembering their mother, a touch on the top of the head reminds them of their father, a touch on the jaw line stimulates feelings about their husband or wife, a touch on the shoulder brings about feelings of brothers/sisters or close friends, and finally, making small circles with the fingertips on the back of the neck brings about feelings of having children. The following photographs show each type of anchored touch.

Each touch must be done within the context of the "conversation." It will be confusing if you are talking about how wonderful it was to be at home with mother and then do the friend

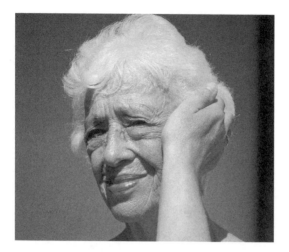

Mother-touch.

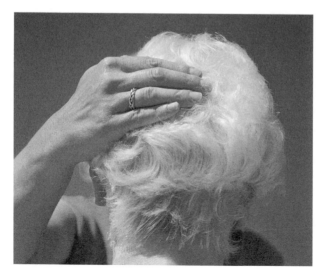

Father-touch.

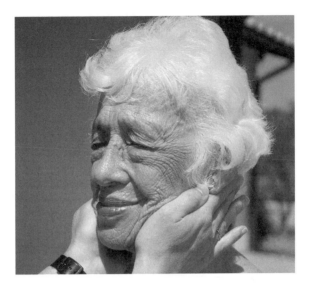

Partner-touch.

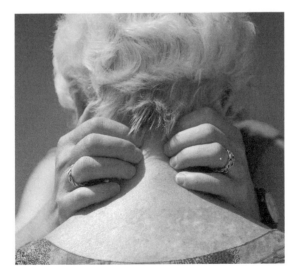

Child-touch.

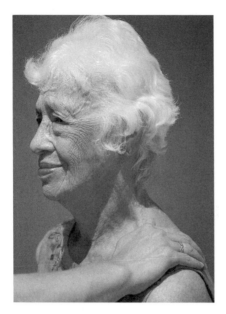

Brother/sister/friend-touch.

touch. There must be congruence between the touch and the subject. Each touch must be done with empathy, feeling the emotion that the other person is feeling, and there must be congruence within yourself. Touch should be used carefully and with great thought and caring.

Using a *clear, warm voice tone* is useful when the conversation is emotionally neutral. Often, people do not realize that their voice tones are harsh, parental, or demeaning. Does your voice typically drop in tone at the end of each sentence? Does it go up? Pay attention to the sound of your voice when you are talking with your disoriented relative. When your relative is expressing emotions, it is important that you match the emotion in your own voice tone. If the person is angry, then you need to reflect the anger; if there is sadness, then your voice should sound sad. Be careful not to "act" or pretend, because it will come out sounding insincere. Instead, match the tone within the context of finding empathy.

Observe the emotion, match the emotion, and say the emotion with emotion. This is useful with people who are expressing feelings in a nonverbal way, such as pounding, pacing, scratching, folding, yelling, or crying. First "calibrate" yourself to your relative. This means that you should observe very carefully, then adjust your body, voice tone, and emotional state to match that of the other person. When you do this with empathy, an emotion will become clear within yourself. At that point, you can simply say what you feel or what you believe the other is feeling.

For example, Mrs. Weber is stomping through the hallway back and forth. When she reaches the end of the hall, she hits the wall, turns, and goes the other way. Her eyes are cast down, her mouth is small with tension, and there is muscle tension in her neck and jaw. Her hands are in loose fists and held into her body. I observe her for a moment and then adjust my face to match hers, I walk next to her in the same rhythm, mirroring the steps and turns (I choose not to hit the wall when she does because that would feel inappropriate or dishonest). The tension I now feel in the neck and jaw reminds me of feeling angry. My voice tone drops, and with anger in my voice I say, "You seem very angry." If I am correct, then Mrs. Weber will look at me and respond. If I am not correct, then she will simply ignore me and continue with what she was doing. I then need to recalibrate and see what I missed or did wrong.

Use *ambiguity* when you do not understand a particular word or phrase. Ambiguity is the use of nonspecific pronouns instead of specific names for things or items. It is a way of focusing on the deeper meaning of what is being said, rather than on the facts. For example,

Mrs. C: "Frand" is gone. (*said sadly, with a worried look on her face*)

  Vicki: It's gone? (*mirroring the look and tone of voice*)
       Where did it go? Is it gone long?

The word "Frand" could be a name or a mispronunciation of "friend." What it is is less important than the feelings that are expressed. One has to explore the feelings and not worry about the facts. Often, one gets caught up in trying to understand and loses sight of the meaning behind what is said.

Linking the behavior to the need works best with disoriented elderly who do not communicate with words and instead use movements to express their needs. Remember the important basic human needs that were considered in Part I:

- Physiological needs for food, drink, shelter, and sexual and sensory stimulation
- The need to feel safe and secure
- The need to be loved and to be affiliated with other people
- The need for recognition and respect from others
- The need to be useful and/or the need for identity involved with working
- The need to make sense of the environment and the people in that environment
- The need for harmony and balance
- The need to resolve unfinished issues before one's death

This technique is another way of trying to connect with the deeper meaning of what is being expressed. For example, Mrs. C. is slowly taking everything out of a drawer. Each item is inspected and laid aside on her bed. She rubs each item firmly. When the drawer is empty, she then slowly puts them back in the drawer one at a time. She is highly concentrated on the task. Her face does not reflect anger, sadness, or pain, just concentration. Mrs. C used to work in a factory on an assembly line, so perhaps she is in "work mode."

Vicki: Is there a lot more to do Mrs. C?
Mrs. C: (*looks up and we have eye contact*)
Vicki: How much more is there to do? Are they in order?

Summary of Techniques for People who Communicate Less Verbally and More Nonverbally

Mirroring

Genuine eye contact

Touch and anchored touch

Clear, warm voice tone

Observe, match, and say the emotion with emotion

Ambiguity

Link the behavior to the need

Music and singing

Use music, not just any music, but the old, familiar songs that your relative enjoyed at various times of her life. The music of youth is particularly imprinted in memory. Very often, disoriented elderly may not be able to speak but can sing the songs of childhood. Some people respond to songs of their teenage years or early adulthood. For a woman who misses her husband, swaying to the sounds of the big bands brings back the warmth of his touch as they danced. Singing together is the best: There is communication and exchange. Learn your relative's favorite songs and sing them with her, even if you have a terrible voice. If classical music was her favorite, then play a recording, but stay with her and perhaps move to the music. Songs can also be used to express emotions. Find a sad song, a happy song, and an angry song and sing them together at appropriate moments. Often, people who have not spoken words in a long time will slowly begin to speak after singing.

Techniques that Work Best with People Who Are in Vegetation

People who are in vegetation do not respond to questions but do respond sometimes to music, touch, and linking the behavior to the need, as described in the previous section. Various forms of sensory stimulation can and should be used. Aromatherapy works beautifully with disoriented elderly who are totally withdrawn, often eliciting strong reactions such as an opening of the eyes, a tear, or movement in the body or hands. Massage not only is good for stimulating circulation and treatment of dry skin but also often is the only way for those in vegetation to receive human contact, to know that someone is there. Again, keep the basic human needs in mind. Any form of sensory stimulation that is done with the needs of the relative always in mind and that is done with caring and love will be a positive thing.

End the Conversation on a Positive Note

Often the conversation will come to a natural end. The problem has been solved for the moment or the emotions have been expressed and relieved. A good ending should lead the way to a new activity or moment.

- "You look like you feel relieved for now. Is that so?"
- "That seems like a good solution."
- "I need to get back to work now, is that okay with you?"

There may be times when the conversation does not come to a natural end, but you need to end it in any case. It is difficult to leave at an emotional moment; however, if you are honest and promise to return, most disoriented older people will accept that.

- "I know you have a lot more to say, but I'm really late and have to go. Can I come back later this afternoon and we can finish this conversation?"

Do not be surprised if your relative does not remember what you were talking about and wants to talk about something entirely different when you return.

When validating people who have clearly expressed a basic human need, you can help that person by supporting her feelings of self-worth:

- "You were a terrific mother."
- "You worked hard all your life."
- "What a caring person you are."
- "You've taught me a lot today."
- "I don't know how you stay so strong."

It is critical that you say these sorts of statements with integrity and honesty. If you do not believe what you are saying, the statement will sound like a lie or condescension. It won't help at all and might break down the trusting relationship you have worked to build. Only say what you really believe, and what will make the older person feel good about herself.

General Points about Using Validation Techniques

You do not need to use all of the techniques, and there is no particular order for using them. The techniques are to help you explore the world of the person with whom you are talking. A good Validation session is like a conversation, with one person being the main focus. Expressing your own feelings or opinions does not necessarily help you communicate better with empathy. Remember your goals: Make contact, communicate, build a trusting relationship, and explore the other person's world.

YOU, TOO, ARE A PERSON: RESPECT YOUR OWN LIMITS, AND ASK FOR HELP

There are times when you cannot or should not use Validation. When your emotions are strong and your own needs are pressing, it will be impossible for you to have empathy. When your mother says, "I want to die"; when your father calls you by your mother's name and treats you like his wife; when your sister says that you have stolen all her money; or when your husband tries to throw you out of the house because he thinks you are a stranger—these are moments when it may be too difficult to put aside your own feelings. Realize that and accept that. The issues will not go away. You will have other moments later to address those complaints in a validating way, but when these first occur, the shock, the hurt, the fear, or the loss may be too immediate to do anything else but have a natural, human reaction. We respond automatically with, "I don't want you to die," "I'm not mother, I'm me," "I didn't steal your money," "I am your wife, don't you recognize me?" These responses may not help the situation, but they may help you to express your feelings. Once the initial response is expressed, you may find yourself thinking, "Well, that didn't help at all. What else could I do?" Perhaps that is the moment when you can take a breath, center yourself, and try to enter your loved one's world. It's not too late.

Caring for a disoriented relative is hard work both physically and psychologically. Learning Validation also is difficult because (for most people) it asks you to integrate a totally new type of behavior and respond with other reflexes. Everyone needs feedback and some supervision as they learn new behavior. Reach out and find someone who can give you help. Contact someone who is trained in Validation to give you advice on handling difficult situations. Sometimes it takes just a word to remind you to center. Sometimes it takes a different approach. Many people find that when they start learning Validation, they become so interested that they wish to go deeper. In that case, it might be interesting for you to take a training course. Resources and contact information are listed in Appendix 4.

Part III

How Validation Works in Real-Life Family Situations

The following stories are real. They are from family members who are or were caring for disoriented relatives and have been able to use Validation to improve their relationship and communication. After each story is a step-by-step guideline for how you can handle similar challenging situations.

Validating is demanding work, and you should not expect to sustain it in every encounter. Do not believe that just because you sometimes cannot transcend your own frustration or are sometimes unable to recognize or understand the reasons for some particular disoriented behavior that you should not practice Validation at all. Each encounter is a unique and specific opportunity to improve communication, build a positive relationship, provide comfort, and acknowledge the humanity of your relative.

Having come this far, you are aware that Validation always involves your willingness and ability to recognize, respect, and relate to what has become another person's reality. Although each of the 10 stories that are told here presents a different situation that leads to a different dialogue, certain fundamentals of the process apply in every case. A reminder of these steps is included in each how-to section.

PREPARING YOURSELF MENTALLY

Part II discussed the need to prepare oneself mentally before starting the Validation process, the steps to take to clear and center. Some people are familiar with this from other contexts—meditation, prayer, yoga, anger management, parenthood—and can readily adapt them to Validation preparation. For others, this will be unfamiliar territory. If you find yourself unable to set your own emotions aside for awhile using these techniques, then you might seek further guidance and take some time to explore them before launching on a Validation encounter.

First, recognize your feelings at the moment (e.g., anger, annoyance, frustration, sadness) and say to yourself, "Not now, later." Your feelings are important and need attention, but they will get in your way and make empathy difficult. Remind yourself that you can handle these feelings later, at a time and a place that are more appropriate. Breathe deeply from your belly, relax your muscles, put your own feelings in the metaphorical closet, and open your heart and mind to your relative (see the centering exercises in Appendix 3).

Set your goal: to explore with respect and love. Sometimes it helps to set yourself a specific goal: "I want to discover who my mother is right now and what is going on in her mind."

OBSERVATION

Once you have prepared yourself, you are ready to shift your focus to the person with whom you wish to make a loving connection. Observing for emotional clues, finding the right distance, and achieving empathy are discussed at some length in Part II, but now that you are considering how to apply these theories to real-life situations, you should review how these steps become part of your process.

Look at your relative's face. What does her facial expression tell you? Is there tension, or is she relaxed? Notice the mouth, eyes, and lips especially. Does she seem to be in a happy state or more worried? Try to match the facial expression. What does the body language tell you? Are the hands tensed? Is the chin jutting out or pulled in? Is she leaning forward? Try to match the level of tension that you observe. What does the voice sound like? Is it high pitched, or is she speaking slowly? Notice the breathing. Is it fast or slow, shallow or deep? Try matching the breathing pattern. When you match, or mirror, the facial expression and the breathing, what emotions come up in you? Try to remember a time when you also felt that way. Put yourself in her shoes; feel what she feels.

As you approach your loved one, try to sense the appropriate distance—the distance where you meet her "boundaries." As you move toward her, be aware of her comfort zone. Notice whether she moves toward you (you are too far away) or leans back a bit with some part of the body (you are too close). Remember that with most people who are in malorientation, you need to keep normal social distance: a handshake distance apart. With individuals who are disoriented, you need to get closer generally. With people who are in repetitive motion and vegetation, you will need to move in very closely, sometimes almost nose to nose, for them to know that you are there. Always be aware of the other's boundaries and needs for closeness or distance. Put aside your own needs for the few moments that you choose to validate. You are now ready to begin.

✻

DORIS AND HER MOTHER: DEALING WITH REPETITION

Mom asks, "What town is this?" just about every 2 minutes on the long car ride from Pennsylvania to her hometown in North

Carolina. She wants to know because she cannot figure out where she is. Her mind is stuck like an old record-player needle in a damaged groove. She wants to know the answer, but she cannot get beyond the question. She cannot record the information so that her mind can play it back to her.

So what should I do? I answer the question, again and again and again. The tension rises in my voice. I know that Mom cannot remember. We are into a 10-hour journey, but it could be 15 minutes or an hour. Mom's conversation is always the same. She wants to know where she is, and I want to tell her, but the communication link is broken. How do I fix it? I joined the Validation family support group at Country Meadows, where Mom lives, to find out. The first thing that I learn is that I cannot fix it. It is broken. I need to figure out how to work with the damaged goods the way they are because Mom is not replaceable. She is not going to change, so I must be more creative, inventive, and patient. I find comfort in knowing that I am not alone. My frustrations are the same as other family members who are dealing with relatives who have dementia. Talking with other families provides a much-needed pressure valve release, but, primarily, I learn that I must look at the world the way Mom does and live in that world with her and work with her limitations.

In this instance, I learned that long car trips are unsuitable for Mom. I also learned that she needs to fill the long silences in a moving car with conversations; Mom needs to be engaged. When I write down our destination on a piece of paper and give it to her, it helps to slow down the number of times she asks, "Where are we?" I can tell her to look for a road sign so that *she* can help me locate where we are.

Have I trained her to behave better? No, I have trained myself. I am practicing Validation. I am accepting Mom's point of view and working from her perspective instead of trying to enforce the more normal social protocols of behavior. I cannot "fix" my mother and must not try, because we both will end up frustrated and angry.

Back in her apartment, Mom wonders if we are in North Carolina. The answer is not a blunt, "No." Instead I ask what she liked best about being raised in North Carolina. I lead her to talk about what she does remember about North Carolina, growing up there, and the people she knew. I am leading her into a comfortable area by using the journalistic "who," "what," "where," "when," and "how" method of collecting information. I find out what she knows, not what she doesn't. Mom lives in a foggy, unclear world, and instead of always trying to remind her of what she cannot see, I must find out what she does see and assure her that she is safe.

WHAT TO DO WHEN YOUR MOTHER REPEATS THE SAME THING OVER AND OVER

The Situation

Mother cannot retain the answer to a question. That answer is important to her because it relates to one of her fundamental needs. She will therefore ask the question every time she experiences the underlying anxiety or need.

The Problem

Understand and accept that the behavior has a reason. It is difficult not to judge her repetitive questioning or get angry, but try to find the reason behind the behavior. Your goal is to get a profound understanding of her reality and accompany your mother within that framework.

A Validation Approach

Step 1: Prepare yourself. Acknowledge and set aside your own feelings, get centered, breathe, relax.

Step 2: Observe. Pay careful attention to facial expression, body language, voice, and breathing. Use mirroring/matching techniques to increase your understanding and find empathy.

Step 3: Explore what your mother is thinking and feeling. Ask questions, and wait for her responses.

Mother: Where are we?
Doris: What looks familiar to you?
Mother: Nothing! Are we lost?
Doris: You look lost. Do you feel lost?
Mother: Absolutely!
Doris: What makes you feel safe?
Mother: Everything is so mixed up. I like it when everything is in order.

Doris: What would help put everything in order?

Mother: If I knew where I was and where we are going.

Doris: Okay, here is the map. Let's track it together.

Doris: When you felt lost or scared in the past, what helped you?

Mother: (*sigh*) I can remember driving with my parents, when we lost our house. Nobody had any money, and we weren't sure where we would live. All the kids were scared. Then my dad started singing songs, and we felt better.

Doris: What songs did you sing?

Mother: Let's see, "My Heart Belongs to Daddy," "God Save America," and "On the Sunny Side of the Street."

Doris: Let's sing together now.

Try to find the connection between what your mother is expressing and one of the basic needs. In this example, it seems that the mother is expressing the need for safety and security. So how can you help her feel more secure? Ask her.

It is great if you can find a solution, but that is not always possible. Sometimes nothing helps. In that case, you need to accept that your mother is scared or lost, and you can only stand by her in a supportive way.

Doris: It's awful to feel scared and lost! (*with lots of empathy*)

By sharing the fear with her, you have helped her feel accepted. She is no longer alone. This could be a moment of intimacy and a time when you can talk about other things.

❄

JOHN ALLEN AND HIS WIFE, JOAN:
WHEN THE PAST BECOMES THE PRESENT

The most difficult thing about visiting my wife in the assisted living facility was that she often did not recognize me. I visited her every day, was consumed with trying to care for her, and struggled to get her to recognize where she was and stop her bizarre behavior. So often she would ask me, "How do I get to the plant from here?" Then there were times when she wanted to see her mother and father. I just didn't know what to say. Every time I gently explained that her parents were dead or that she didn't work any more, she would stop talking, close her eyes, and drop her head. She shut me out. So often I would find her walking the hallway as though she were checking the production line. She used to work in a factory and did that kind of thing. When our son came to visit, she didn't recognize him either, or she would talk with him as though she were talking to a friend, her brother, or even her father. He didn't know how to handle that either. It was frustrating to say the least. We didn't want to stop visiting her, but it didn't seem to do any good for anyone.

My son and I were invited to join the facility's family support group and were introduced to Validation. We went every week, and after awhile began to see the meaning of what Joan was doing. Her behavior was not so bizarre. It came from a deep need to be useful, to be productive, and to be secure again. The most difficult thing for my son and me was to really accept that Joan was never going to be the woman she was before she became disoriented and to embrace her as she is now. We had to step into her reality and walk alongside her. My son and I learned things about my wife that we never knew. We learned about her life before we got married, her dream of being a singer and going to New York to pursue it, and, like so many others of our generation, having a war put an end to that dream. Joan went to work in a factory to do her part to "help our boys over there." My son learned how becoming a mother was one of the greatest joys of her life, how his birth and existence in her life changed her in ways that she never dreamed possible. I think my son actually felt closer to his mother than ever before.

For me, learning this way of being with my wife after so many years changed me as well. Like most men, I never talked about feelings, but by accepting her as she is, I found out how much Joan gave up to be with me. She told me that throughout our years together, she saw me as her knight in shining armor, even though I fell from my steed many times. I was able to see the

20-year-old girl I fell in love with, still there in this 86-year-old woman. By traveling with her into the past, I found a way to be with her in the present.

HOW TO REACT WHEN YOUR WIFE THINKS THAT IT IS 1942

The Situation

Joan has mentally returned to a time when she felt most productive and useful.

The Problem

It can be shocking, disappointing, and hurtful to see your wife in a state of time confusion. We want our loved ones to be like they were. It is difficult to accept the changes that disorientation brings.

A Validation Approach

Step 1: Prepare yourself. Surprise often is the first reaction, followed by sadness, and that is a normal, human response. However, if you want to build a better relationship and communicate with her, then this reaction will not help, so you need to center yourself and put away your own feelings for the moment.

Step 2: Observe your wife carefully. What is she doing? When you match or mirror the facial expression and the breathing, which emotions do you sense in her?

Step 3: Explore your wife's personal reality by asking questions. Your goal should be to find out what is going on and what is important to her at that moment.

Joan: How do I get to the plant from here?

John: What do you do at the plant?

Joan: You know, I have to check the line. There's a lot.

John: A lot of work. Did you also have a lot of fun?

Joan: Oh my, yes. All my friends are there, and we lunch together. Of course we always think about the boys at the front. We try to do our best for the war effort.

John: You always did really good work. What was it like then?

Joan: Oh, we had such a good time. I'd go down the line every morning, and the girls and I would have lunch together in the lunchroom. After work, we'd wave good-bye. "See you tomorrow." You know, we had the best production figures of all. That's 'cause we knew what we were doing and why.

John: What was the best thing?

Joan: Feeling a part of something important.

John: I know you were. It must have been wonderful. It's time for me to go, but I'll see you tomorrow, okay?

Joan: Lovely dear. See you tomorrow.

———————

Try to recognize the underlying need or emotion that your wife is expressing. In this dialogue, the wife is expressing several different things: the need to be productive, the need to be a part of a group of people, and, emotionally, she seems to be expressing pride in her work. It is good to reinforce that feeling by saying something such as, "You do good work," but only if you really say it with honesty. Do not feel as though you have to come to a special or significant ending. When you have to go or you feel that her energy is getting lower, then it is time to stop. Try to end the conversation on a positive note if it is possible.

Your wife has gone back to 1942 for a very good reason: that period of her life held feelings that she is missing today. Do not concentrate so much on the time confusion; instead, concentrate on the feelings and needs. Share those with her, and you will find a meeting place where you can enjoy being together.

✳

NANCY AND HER MOTHER: ENTERING YOUR MOTHER'S WORLD

My mother was so suspicious of everyone, including me. It seemed that after we had to sell her home and put her in an assisted living facility, she couldn't trust anyone. She walked around with her purse stuffed with things such as jewelry and hankies. Every time I visited, she would ask the same question over and over, "Where is my house?" and complain that Shirley, an old friend, was constantly taking her things. I wanted her to stop. I got so frustrated with her; I hated to visit her. She got really angry with me, to the point of shouting, when I would try to tell her that we had to sell her home or say, "Mom, Shirley isn't stealing your things, she is dead." I would leave in tears. A staff member encouraged me to attend a family support meeting. It was comforting because I discovered that I wasn't alone. I learned a new way of dealing with my mother. I realized that her behavior had a reason behind it and that my mother's anger stemmed from many life losses. I began to say things such as, "Mom, who takes your things?" "What things do they take?" "Have other things been taken from you?" "Are there times when they don't take things?" This approach seemed to work for both of us. She wasn't as angry, and I wasn't as frustrated. The staff where my mother lives noticed that she was a lot calmer after our visits; she was even pleasant. I don't always understand everything she talks about, but I work hard at not letting her know that. This has made all the difference.

LETTING GO AND ENTERING YOUR MOTHER'S WORLD

The Situation

This example clearly shows the clash of two opposite sets of needs. Nancy wants to have a "normal" mother, a mother who is not in malorientation. The mother's need seems to be to express anger about all of her losses and perhaps to deny them.

The Problem

Your mother cannot change, so if there is to be some sort of positive relationship between the two of you, then you will have to be the one to adapt. Although it may be difficult, you need to let go of your expectations, let go of the wishes, and instead open yourself up to who your mother is at this moment. Your feelings and needs are real and important but can better be expressed with a friend, a partner, or a counselor—someone who can listen to you and respond with empathy. Your mother cannot do this.

A Validation Approach

Step 1: Center yourself. Breathe. Clear away the emotions (frustration, anger, sadness). This takes practice and is not always easy to do.

Step 2: Observe your mother carefully; calibrate.

Step 3: Explore your mother's world by asking her about it. Set your goal: Find out what is bothering her.

Mother: Where is my house?

Nancy: Do you miss your house?

Mother: Of course I do. I've had that house for 35 years. They took it away from me.

Nancy: What do you miss the most?

Mother: Well, just having it.

Nancy: You miss being a homeowner.

Mother: Exactly. People just take things that don't belong to them. It's not right.

Nancy: What else are you missing?

Mother: Shirley took my things.

Nancy: What things are gone?

Mother: My mother's jewelry, which she gave me before she died, is missing and all my lovely monogrammed hand-kerchiefs. I had lovely, delicate handkerchiefs—all gone.

Nancy: All gone! Tell me about the jewelry. What were your favorite pieces?

Mother: There was an elegant brooch with a small emerald in it, it was gold. That was my favorite. (*she sighs as the anger fades into sadness*)

Nancy: You have lost so much. That is so sad.

Mother: I've had hard times, but I'm glad you're here now. Tell me, what's going on with the children?

––––––––––––––

Remember, you cannot get her house back or get her to acknowledge that time has been the thief that took the things about which she cared. The best thing that you can do is to have empathy with her sense of loss and share that feeling. Realize that she might always need to talk about her house and her jewelry before moving on to other subjects. Prepare yourself for that. When you acknowledge and validate her sense of loss, she will be more likely to move on. She has lost a lot. That is real. It is not difficult to have empathy with that, because we have all suffered losses and know that sadness.

Children often are faced with the burden of selling the family house when parents can no longer maintain it. This can be a no-win situation. The parents lose not only their house but also, sometimes more important, their status as a homeowner, and with that, their independence. In one move, they become dependent, old, powerless, and at the end of the line with no recourse or reprieve. You may feel guilty about having sold the prized house and, without realizing it, be trying to get your parents to forgive you, because if the parents accept the sale and the situation, then you are absolved of guilt. It is important to recognize whether this is going on. The goal now is to create a positive relationship, build communication, and share the last years of your parents' lives with some pleasure and, hopefully, love.

❅

MRS. PRACHEL AND HER MOTHER: RESPECTING THE ADULT

I've been caring for my mother for the past 5 years at home, where we live together. I moved in when it became impossible for her to care for herself. She was 83 then. My 20 years of nursing experience has certainly helped but didn't really prepare me for how hard it is, day in and day out, to deal with the emotional pressures. Sometimes mother forgets who I am and why I'm there. She starts shouting at me to get out and leave her alone. She needs help bathing, going to the toilet, getting dressed, preparing meals, taking her medications, and, well, just about everything. She has no sense of time or season, not recognizing when it's cold or hot outside. One time she started singing Christmas songs in the middle of summer. My way of dealing with her was to stay calm and treat her like any patient. I spoke calmly, gently correcting her when she said something wrong or out of place. I tried to be kind, to care for her, like she cared for me when I was young. It got to the point when my patience was wearing thin. I couldn't sleep well at night from worry. I stopped going out anywhere with friends and was too embarrassed to invite friends to our home. My entire life was centered on mother, and that was becoming an unbearable weight to carry around my neck.

I was looking on the Internet and came across an article on Validation, which got me interested. After reading the book, I tried a few of the techniques described, and they would sometimes work, but often there was no difference at all in how my mother behaved. I read about a support group for family members who take care of disoriented relatives. I had never been the sort of person who would join such a group, but I really was at the end of my rope, so I joined, thinking that if I didn't feel comfortable, then I would not continue. The thing that struck me the most was how similar everyone felt. Many of the people had the same sorts of problems and were as frustrated and helpless as I was. The group leader was a nurse who had as many years of experience as I did and was trained in Validation. She was great and was able to help us all see our relatives with different eyes. I finally realized that I had to stop trying to change my mother, to correct her all the time. I had to let go. The other thing that was difficult for me to understand was that expressing emotions is a good thing for my mother, not something that would make our lives together more difficult. I'm not an emotional person, but I can understand that because my mother can't control herself anymore, her emotions spill out. I can see that when she expresses a lot of feelings, such as anger or sadness, she feels better afterward. That's better. When she forgets who I am, I no longer see that as a slap in the face but realize that she may be using me as a symbol for someone from her past. I try to ask her questions such as, "When did that happen before?" exploring what she is talking about instead of trying to correct her. The techniques seemed silly in the beginning, and I had difficulty just asking questions. It took awhile to get comfortable with it all. Looking back now, I can see a huge difference at home. Mother and I get along much better, mainly because I've stopped pushing her to accept my reality and correcting her. She gets less angry at me, and there is more peace. We've actually had some great talks about her past, and I've found out a lot of things I never knew.

REALIZE THAT MOTHER HAS NOT BECOME A CHILD

The Situation

When your mother becomes disoriented, you can feel hurt, sad, and angry, and it is certainly a huge loss. One way of handling these feelings is to bury them under a desire to help, to make it better, or to get control of the situation. This creates distance from the unpleasant feelings. It also creates distance with your mother because it denies her needs and feelings. Often people in helping professions (e.g., nurses, teachers, other caregivers) get caught up in the "helper mentality." This sets up a hierarchical relationship, with the patient/student/disoriented parent at the receiving end and you in the position of strength. An adult-to-adult relationship is better for building trust and enhancing communication. Although it may feel as though your mother is a child because she has lost social controls or orientation to time, she is an adult with a lifetime of experience, memories, and wisdom. She needs to be respected and treated like an adult.

The Problem

You may not realize that you are treating your disoriented mother like a child. Try to hear your own voice tone. Often, that is the strongest clue. Do you use a "teacher voice"? Try taping yourself talking with your mother if you cannot hear it and you suspect that you are doing this. Pay attention to the words that you use. Do you use the word "we" instead of "you," as in, "Shall we go to the bathroom?" Do you feel as though you are controlling yourself all the time? Is there tension in your chest or throat? These are some of the clues to look for.

A Validation Approach

Step 1: Center yourself. Set your goal: to explore with respect and love. Breathe deeply.

Step 2: Observe your mother carefully. What is she doing? How is she doing it? Which emotions are being expressed? Use matching and mirroring.

Step 3: Begin a conversation with your mother with the goal of sharing her emotions.

Mother:	Get out! Leave me alone!
Nancy:	What do you want to do?
Mother:	I want to take care of myself!
Nancy:	What is the worst thing about someone taking care of you?
Mother:	I don't like the messing about. Messy, messy, messy. Dressy, dressy, dressy.
Nancy:	What gets so messy?
Mother:	The children need to be cleaned and washed and dressy, dressy, dressy.
Nancy:	You took such good care of your children. Do you miss that?
Mother:	I love my children. See, there's one, two, three. We need to get them ready now. (*singing*) The itsy, bitsy spider crawled up the water spout.
Together:	(*singing*) Down came the rain and washed the spider out. Out came the sun and dried up all the rain; and the itsy, bitsy spider crawled up the spout again.
Nancy:	I remember you singing that to me all the time. Do you want to get cleaned up now?

Do not worry about the logic of your conversation. If you can share feelings and communicate with her, then you have been successful. This mother wants to feel useful, to take care of her children. When she is treated like a child, she cannot fulfill that need. You can join her, accept her as she is, and enjoy the warmth of her mothering.

❋

JILL AND HER GRANDMOTHER: HELPING YOUNG PEOPLE RELATE

My name is Jill, and my grandmother was told by her doctors that she has Alzheimer's disease. I am 13 years old. My grandmother is 78 years old. My grandmom used to be a lot of fun to be around. We'd go shopping and she'd let me buy really cool stuff. Sometimes my mom got mad at us, but Grandmom would just say, "Hey, remember when you were young." I remember that my grand-mom started doing things that were really strange. One time she forgot to pick me up from school. She just never showed up and got really angry when my mom questioned her about it. She tried to blame my mom for her mistake. One time when we were shopping, she got really mad at the store people because they laughed at her. She had asked for a Christmas book and it was June. More and more things like that began to happen. My grandmother became scary because she got mad really easily. One day I was with her and she accused me of taking a ring that my grandfather gave her. She yelled at me and said bad things. I began to cry and didn't want to be around her. I never knew what she would do.

My mother and I went to classes to help us understand my grandmother better. It helped to understand how I was feeling about what was happening to me because of my grandmother's illness. One thing I really liked was learning how to "center," or relax. It helped to calm me down and know that I was fine. It seemed to be easier for me to do that than for my mom. I could listen to my grandmom better, even when she was angry. I stopped thinking she was mad at me and learned how to talk with her when she was angry.

My grandmother has this thing about people stealing her things. She accuses everyone. I learned that some of that may come from her past. When she was younger, her family became very poor during the Depression. My grandmother probably realizes the loss of her memory, and to her it feels like she is being robbed. I learned that it was better asking her, "What did they take?" "When did they take these things?" "Where did they take these things?" When I asked her these questions, she didn't get as mad as when I used to try to tell her that no one was taking these things. I felt more comfortable knowing how to handle these situations. She may still get mad for awhile, but then she gets over it and is nice again. My visits with her are better.

TEACHING YOUNG PEOPLE TO RELATE WITH DISORIENTED OR MALORIENTED GRANDPARENTS

The Situation

Jill is scared by and can't understand Grandmom's disoriented behavior. What once was a warm and loving relationship has become fraught with fear and insecurity. From the grandmother's perspective, she is using her granddaughter as a symbol for people from her past and expressing pent-up emotions about past events.

The Problem

Jill needs the most help with understanding the situation and setting up her expectations for moments of contact. To develop a positive relationship between grandmother and granddaughter, Jill needs to accept that Grandmom cannot do what she used to do. She needs help finding alternative ways of being with her and reacting to her behavior.

A Validation Approach

Step 1: As Jill says in her story, younger people often find relaxation and centering easy to do.

Step 2: Although observation has always been the next step in the process of validating, in such a situation, an adult needs to do the observation and then translate that information to the child. She needs information about Grandmom's behavior. Depending on the age of the grandchild, you should explain a bit about malorientation and disorientation. With older children, such as Jill, you can offer a more complex explanation. With younger children, keep it simple. It is important to use positive phrasing rather than negative images. Do not say, "Grandma is crazy now"; instead, you should explain, "Grandma is in the last part of her life. She is forgetful because her brain isn't working as well as before. Sometimes she makes mistakes with time, like when she thought it was Christmas and it was really summertime. There is nothing that we can do to make it better; we just have to accept it." Adding personal information that helps explain the unusual behavior is important. "Grandma had a difficult life. When she was a girl, around your age, there was a Depression. Lots of people lost all their money and their jobs. Grandma's father lost his job, and so the family had to move out of their house. That was an awful experience. Grandma was really poor for a long time, and the family struggled to get through it. When she was older, things got better, but I don't think she ever forgot those hard times. She learned to be very careful with money and her things. So now, when she is missing something and she doesn't remember where she put her purse, for instance, she will complain that someone stole it. She feels like she was robbed, just like she felt that everything was taken from her when she was a girl."

Step 3: Help the grandchild to develop specific ways of reacting to situations that arise regularly. "When Grandma is confused in time, like when she asked for Christmas books, here is what you can do: First, breathe and relax; look at her, and ask her, 'What's going on?' Listen to her answer, and try to really understand what is going on in her mind. Ask questions such as, 'When did that happen before?' 'What reminds you of that?' 'What was it like when you were my age?' When Grandma gets angry at you, first breathe and try to relax; remember that she is mostly angry about getting older, not at you. Ask her, 'What made you so angry?' Really listen to her answer."

Here are simple dos and don'ts to follow:

- Never correct Grandma or tell her that she is wrong.

- Try to stay centered and not get frustrated or angry.

- Really listen and focus on her world, her reality. Find out what is going on.

- Try to learn something about Grandma's life. Like all older people, she has been through a lot in her life and has very interesting stories to tell. You can learn from her.

Developing a positive relationship between grandmother and granddaughter is the goal. Sharing old stories and finding the moments of loving contact are the building blocks. Together, they can create a relationship that is fulfilling for both.

Another positive outcome of satisfying contact between the grandchild and the grandmother is that the young person can learn to approach old age without fear and with acceptance. How she learns to deal with her grandmother is the beginning of learning how to deal with her own aging process. Although this may seem a long way off in the future, the lessons that she learns now will stay with her for the rest of her life. As a parent, please recognize that the attitudes that you teach your child most likely are the attitudes that she will carry with her as she gets older. A positive attitude toward aging will help her to accept her own losses and gains as she goes through life.

MAX AND HIS "WAITING FOR JOHNNIE" MOTHER: ACCEPTING HER THE WAY SHE IS

Coming to visit my mother was difficult, especially for me, the oldest son. She always had this lost look about her. The staff where she resides tells me that she's pleasant but very reluctant to engage in any activities. She sits all day on a bench near her room, pocketbook in hand. She tells people who stop to say hello, "I'm waiting for my Johnnie to come home." John is my father. He died 2 years ago from cancer. He cared for my mother at home until the very end. My sister and I knew we needed to be there more, but our dad insisted that they were fine. Mother has always been so full of life and fun. Now . . . she just sits. All of our encouragement could not spark interest in anything. "No, I need to be here when Johnnie comes home. He loves to see me when he gets off his ship. I can't miss him." My father was a career Navy man. My mother spent most of her days waiting for dad. I felt so guilty saying things like, "Dad's ship is delayed and he wants you to come home," or, "Mom, dad won't be coming home." It seemed to make her more uneasy and even irritable.

One day I came to visit earlier than usual. I happened to hear a conversation that my mother was having with a staff member, who talked to my mother as though they were best friends. She asked questions such as, "Is he usually on time?" "Has he ever been late?" "How much do you miss him?" "What do you miss most about him?" I was fascinated and surprised at how well my mother handled this dialogue. "Where did you meet Johnnie?"

"What do you love most about him?" "How difficult is it now when he is not here?" With this, my mother cried and revealed her loneliness. Then she looked at the staff member as clear as day and said, "Johnnie really isn't coming home, you know." The staff member just held her hand, just for a moment. My mom seemed alright with that. I talked with this staff member later and started to attend a family support group to learn about Validation. I began to relax around my mother and engaged her in conversation about what she needed. I learned to cry with her, laugh with her, or just sit and be silent with her. My mother loved music. I grew comfortable singing and humming some of the songs that I remembered she loved. I even learned to dance with her, which helped me keep the connection with her when she began losing her language skills. My mother has since passed away, but some of my fondest memories are the ones we had over the last few months of her life.

ACCEPTING YOUR MOTHER, JUST AS SHE IS

The Situation

Your mother is expressing her need for love and her husband by waiting for him, as she frequently did in the past. She has not accepted the reality of living in a nursing facility and does not want to conform to the wishes of those around her, including her children.

The Problem

The son is having difficulty accepting his mother's disorientation. It can be painful, shocking, scary, or simply terribly sad to see one's mother no longer aware of reality. This is one of the most difficult issues that the children of disoriented parents face, but face it they must and, hopefully, come to grips with the loss. The son needs to recognize that the problem lies with his expectations, not with his mother. He needs to accept her, just as she is, before entering a supportive and loving relationship.

A Validation Approach

Before beginning to validate, it is important first to find a new way of looking at the situation. Instead of viewing your mother's behavior through the lens of your own norms and values, try to see it from other perspectives. Here are a few things to consider.

One of the fascinating things about validating people who are in time confusion is when they demonstrate awareness of several levels of consciousness at the same time. Max's mother knew that her husband was dead, yet said that she was waiting for him. This is the reason that she did not react positively when Max said, "He's delayed." He might have been trying to make her feel better, but she knew that what he said was not true.

Max's mother seems perfectly happy to sit and wait for her husband. She may be disoriented and in time confusion, but she also seems relatively happy in that state of being. Of course, she feels loneliness at times. She has lost her life partner, a man who was the center of her life. She will not get over that loss. She cannot replace him; she does not want to replace him. She wants to keep him and his memory close to her, so she does what she has always done: wait for his ship to come in and for him to come home.

Step 1: Use centering to help you clear away the thoughts and feelings. Recognize that this means that you have to acknowledge the loss of the mother you once had. This is significant and sometimes very difficult to do. Set yourself a specific goal: "I want to discover who my mother is right now and what is going on in her mind."

Step 2: Observe your mother carefully. Try to find empathy to experience in yourself the emotion that she is experiencing.

Step 3: Explore your mother's world, and try to be there with her.

Max:	Hi, mom. How are you?
Mother:	Oh, hello. I'm waiting for Johnnie to get back.
Max:	Have you been waiting long?
Mother:	Oh yes, but he always comes home to me, and he loves to see me after such a long trip.
Max:	Do you miss him when he's gone?
Mother:	Of course.
Max:	What do you miss the most?
Mother:	I'm so alone. He's so strong. He holds my hand, and we look at each other.
Max:	Is it that you feel safe with him?
Mother:	Safe and warm and whole.

Max: Whole! Did he complete you?

Mother: That's it. It's not easy bringing up children all alone and taking care of everything, you know.

Max: I know. You did a great job with us. What was that old song you sang with Dad all the time? "Let me call you Sweetheart." (*mother and son sing together*)

By singing together, Max can bring back his mother's feelings of being safe and warm and whole. Dancing together can do this as well. This is the need that seems to come out the strongest in this conversation. The son could also explore the theme of bringing up children all alone and the difficulties that she experienced, if that seems to engage her.

Spending the last part of your mother's life in close, loving contact is a gift for both of you. It can be healing; it can be a satisfying closure of issues that were never resolved. It can make for a more peaceful ending when your mother eventually dies. Accepting your mother, even in a state of time confusion, will open doors to another level of relating. You have much to gain, as does your mother.

❋

EMILY AND HER HUSBAND, SAMUEL: NOT BEING RECOGNIZED

Sam and I got married when he was 25 years old and I was just 23. He's now 82 years old, and I remember that day, 57 years ago, so clearly. He held me close and said that we would never be apart. Later, when he had a chance to take a job that would have paid him a fantastic salary, he turned it down because he would have had to travel a lot. We never had children, but then we felt our life together was complete as it was, together and very happy.

It's important to know that background to understand how totally unprepared I was and unable to cope with Sam's behavior when he developed Alzheimer's disease. He forgot who I was. Sometimes he would remember after a gentle reminder, and sometimes he wouldn't. I would shout, "Sam, it's me, Emily, your wife!" I cried more during those times than ever before. What brought the whole thing to a crisis was what happened one evening 5 years ago. I came home from my monthly women's club meeting at around 9 P.M., and when Sam saw me, he started shouting, "Get out of my house! What would my wife say if I let a strange woman into our house? Get out!" I answered, "But, Sam, I am your wife! It's me, Emily!" I was frantic. The look in his eye was so far away, in another world, and I had no idea how to connect. He shoved me out the door and locked it. As I stood on the stoop of the house that we had shared for so many years, I lost it. I sat down and cried on the steps, not knowing what to do or to whom to turn. After a half hour, I went to the back door and let myself in again. This time Sam recognized me after a minute, and the rest of the evening went fine.

A friend of mine at the women's club had told me about Validation and got the book for me as a gift. I heard that Naomi Feil, the woman who started Validation, was going to give a lecture, so I signed up for it. It was enlightening, to say the least. I came out of that workshop with a feeling of hope. Although I could not change the course of the illness that Sam has, I could change the way I react to him. I had to see things from his perspective, rather than try to convince him that my point was right. The next time Sam didn't recognize me, I simply didn't argue. That was difficult, but it worked. Once I felt okay about not jumping in to defend myself, I started to ask simple questions, such as, "When will your wife come home?" or "What does she look like?" To that question, Sam began to describe me in the most wonderful way. It felt so good to hear that he really does love me. By the end of his description, I could see that he recognized me again. He took my hands and kissed my forehead. We both had tears in our eyes. I don't know how Sam's illness will progress or what other difficulties we will face, but for now, I feel like I can handle it.

THE AGONY OF NOT BEING RECOGNIZED

The Situation

There is probably no worse situation than not being recognized by a disoriented relative. When your mother, father, or husband does not know who you are, it can feel like a blow. It can feel like a stripping of your identity. It can be disorienting for you. The normal rules of social behavior are suddenly suspended, and your personal history feels as though it is erased. You might think, "Well if my husband doesn't know who I am, then what's the point of doing anything for him?" Know that on some level your husband does know who you are. Your history with him is still there. You are still you. He has other things going on at those moments of no recognition, things that may have nothing to do with you, things from his past. You may be a symbol, representing someone else.

From Samuel's perspective, the situation is different. Samuel is seeking his wife with brown hair, the wife he married, the wife who looks like she did many years ago. He does not recognize a white-haired, older woman. He does not see himself as older because his reality is connected to the past. Imagine what it might feel like from his perspective. He knows on some level that he is dependent on his wife. Without her, he is lost. In comes this strange woman. Now he is lost and in a scary situation that has potential danger. His reaction is to push the scary person away and defend himself.

The Problem

Samuel needs time to make the connection between the past and the present and to get through the panic of not recognizing his wife. Emily can help him by remaining calm and trying to engage him in conversation. He will recognize a tone of voice, a touch, her eyes, or maybe a smile. Finding the connecting path to him is not straight, and it does not go through logic or reason. Emily needs to find the emotional path.

A Validation Approach

Step 1: Allow your understanding of the situation to help alleviate some of the pain. Put it in perspective. Practice the centering techniques a lot. To get through those difficult situations, you need to put your feelings aside for a little while. It is crucial for you to have another place to express your feelings—but not with your husband at those moments. Train yourself to breathe, relax, and think about what could be going on in your husband to create such a reaction. Start to focus on his feelings and needs, rather than on your feelings and needs.

Step 2: Observe him carefully. Sometimes focusing on very specific physical characteristics can help you gain objectivity. Try to find the characteristics that he typically demonstrates during these moments of no recognition. If you can identify the physical changes that occur when your husband is in this mindset, then you can recognize this state in the future and not be as surprised by his lack of recognition.

Step 3: Explore what is going on in your husband's world by asking questions. It is very important that you be respectful and engaged in his emotions. If you can have empathy with him, then it is even better.

Samuel:	What are you doing? Who are you?
Emily:	Who are you expecting?
Samuel:	My wife will be home any minute. You better get out of here before she comes.
Emily:	What does she look like?
Samuel:	She has wavy, dark hair and brown eyes. She's not too tall. She comes up to here on me.
Emily:	What do you like the best about her?
Samuel:	She's so soft and gentle. She cares for me. She's there for me.
Emily:	Does she always come home to you?
Samuel:	Always. We are always together. Always have been.
Emily:	She's always there for you. What would happen if she wasn't there?
Samuel:	That would be terrifying. I couldn't take that.
Emily:	Would you feel lost and lonely?
Samuel:	That's right.
Emily:	(*seeing recognition in his eyes and touching his face*) I'm here now.
Samuel:	So you are. Time for a cup of tea.

This is exactly the sort of situation in which an anchor can be useful. An anchor is a connection between a sensory experience and an emotion. (See the discussion of anchors in Part I.) If you can make a connection between a touch and feeling loving/safe, then you can use that anchor when your husband does not recognize you or is scared and lost. You would use the anchor within the context of a conversation such as in the preceding dialogue. An anchor works best once the intensity of the initial emotion has been expressed, so do not start with the anchor. First talk, and then use the anchor.

Finding the different ways of making a connection with your husband can be satisfying. Letting go of your expectations can be freeing. Even within this very difficult situation, there are ways to view and handle it in a positive, constructive way. There can be moments of joy and moments when you share your love. These moments can give you strength to get through the difficult times.

❀

HELEN AND HER SISTER, MERYL: WANTING TO GO HOME NOW!

Meryl is my sister, and she has Alzheimer's disease. My name is Helen. Meryl was 17 years old when I was born. All my life, she was bigger than life to me. When our mother died, Meryl filled her shoes, stepped right into them without blinking an eye. Now, at 79 years old, I see her struggling with simple things. My sister gets lost in her own thoughts.

Her friends and neighbors began to notice changes in her far earlier than I did, but there comes a time when you can't hide from it anymore. For me, the realization began when my sister could not figure out simple things, such as why a light bulb wouldn't work anymore, or when she locked herself out of the house repeatedly. The neighbor family would find her outside at all hours of the night. The hardest thing that I ever had to do was move her from her home to an assisted living facility. She was so angry with me. Our visits were hard. She wanted me to take her home. She begged me not to have her locked up. I didn't know what to do. I tried to tell her that we just needed to fix up her house, but lying to her just didn't feel right to me, and she seemed to know that it was a lie. I would tell her that I would take her home in a few days, and that seemed to quiet her down for a while. I knew that it was wrong to do that, but what else was I suppose to do?

One day, a neighbor called and said that my sister was standing in front of her home. She had somehow gotten out of the facility. It took a lot of convincing to get her into the car, but eventually she did. I took her back to the place she hated, a place where she felt abandoned, a place to escape from, and a place where security became a priority. That was devastating to Meryl and me. I felt that I had betrayed the one person in the world who had always been in my corner. I was a mess!

Understanding and help came in the form of a support group at the facility where my sister was living. I learned how to deal more effectively with my sister's behavior. I learned to listen and to be with her in her pain and sadness. I never realized that she had lost so many things and had so much sadness. The sadness of losing her home, a home that she loved, was stronger than I had imagined. The fear of not always remembering, of losing her mind, plagued her. The confusion of not knowing where she fit in life was something that made me think about my own aging. Sometimes we sat in silence; I learned to be quiet. We talked a lot about many things. One thing I enjoyed were my sister's memories of our mother and father. It was enriching for both of us. We talked like we had not often talked before. I could listen better to all that she had to say, and, oh boy, did she have lots of things to say. She continues to want to go home and I can accept that she always will, but I can handle that better. I know one day she won't ask to go home anymore . . . she won't be doing anything anymore. Her challenging questions will just become a bittersweet memory for me. I learned that even in all of her confusion, she is and always will be my big sister.

HOW TO HANDLE, "I WANT TO GO HOME NOW!"

The Situation

Meryl is desperately trying to go home because she wants to feel safe, secure, independent, and healthy. These are some of the feelings or needs that are associated with being at home. Every person has his or her unique associations with home. A home can be a symbol for adulthood, for having worth or status, or even identity. The home where a person has lived for most of his or her life is a lot more than just a building or an address. Helen is feeling stuck, frustrated, guilty, and despairing because she had no choice but to move her sister into the institution.

The Problem

Moving a loved one from her home to an institution often is emotionally complex for the person who makes the decision. You can feel guilty about it even though you know that it is the best solution for the situation. This guilt can be expressed unconsciously, for instance by trying over and over again to get the relative to accept and enjoy her new surroundings or by denying her angry rejection of the institution. It is too difficult for Helen to open herself up to and accept Meryl's expression of feelings because her own feelings are pressing.

A Validation Approach

Step 1: When your sister says, "I have to go home now," you first need to center yourself. Clear away your own feelings. Remind yourself that the goal of this moment of contact is to build a loving, trusting relationship with your sister and to help her to express her feelings and needs. It is particularly important for you to come back to your feelings after the Validation session. Try to deal with them outside your relationship with your sister. She cannot help you directly. She may not be able to listen to your feelings. She is wrapped up in her own world; she is struggling with her own unresolved issues. Find a place, a person, or a group that can support you.

Step 2: Observe your sister, knowing that this will help you in at least two ways: It will help you focus on something objective, and it will give you clues as to what is going on in your sister's mind.

Step 3: Begin to explore her world.

Meryl: I have to go home right now!

Helen: What's going on?

Meryl: I'm locked up here and can't get out. I don't want to be here. I need to get out of here. Help me! You've locked me up. Get me out of here!

Helen: What's the worst thing about being here?

Meryl: Everything here is bad. The people are crazy. Those nurses don't care at all. I can't find anything. I don't belong here.

Helen: Where do you belong?

Meryl: Home: 86 Willow Street.

Helen: What do you love most about the house on Willow Street?

Meryl: It's where I belong, where my things are, where I take care of everyone.

Helen: You belong in that house. You took care of everyone your whole life.

Meryl: That's right. When mother passed, when the others left, when dad passed, I was there. I am always there.

Helen: You were a rock that we all held onto. What would we have done without you?

Meryl: You were always a good girl. You never got into trouble like Billy. But you were so delicate. I always worried about you getting hurt. Remember when Martha bullied you at school and I had to go in to talk to the principal?

Helen: No, I don't remember. Tell me about that.

Meryl: Martha had made fun of you on your way home from lunch one day. It was springtime, I think. At any rate, you came home from lunch scared that she would beat you up or something. After lunch I walked back to school with you and had a good talk to Martha and then went right into the principal's office and told him that he had to do something about that girl.

Helen: You were a great protector! I remember. Meryl, thank you for taking such good care of me back then.

(The two women sit quietly, holding hands and smiling.)

In the preceding dialogue, Meryl's need to be seen as "in charge," as a protector, is supported. This is a key theme for her. With this support for her identity, she can let go of the immediate need "to go home." You have found a lovely way to share some memories and help her feel more worthwhile.

❋

SARA AND HER MOM: LYING AND PLAY-ACTING

My name is Sara. My mom and I worked together for 25 years running our family business. I started when I was 18 years old, working with both parents every day. My father died of cancer 10 years ago. Since that time, it has just been my mom and me.

My mother has always been very independent, strong, and a very good businesswoman. I remember my dad telling people that if it hadn't been for Mom's good business sense, their furniture business would have failed many times. So, of course, a couple of years ago, I didn't want to believe some of the things that I began to see my mother do: Accounts were messed up, deliveries were wrong, and bills were not being paid. One Sunday morning, she called me to say that I was late for work. We were never open on Sundays. When I told her this, she got angry with me and tried to tell me that it was Monday morning. When I went down to the store, I found her just sitting in the office like a lost soul. It frightened me, particularly when I realized that she had driven herself to work. We had a terrible fight when I insisted on driving her home. "I'm not stupid," she said, "I raised you, MISSY . . . you are not raising me." I followed her home, and she did alright. I don't think she even knew that I was behind her. She got out of her car, went into the house, and never turned the car off. It was in the garage with the door closed and running. Again, when I confronted her and showed her what she had done, she got angry and tried to say that I was trying to make her look crazy. She even accused me of turning the car on to make her look bad.

My story may not be like others. We were lucky. My mother's younger sister is a Mercy Nun, and her order allowed her to move home with Mom to take care of her. She has been a Godsend, no pun intended. As time went on, my mom was more and more difficult to handle. Her confusion would often make her very anxious, and she was quite persistent in claiming that her perceptions of reality were true. She often would get dressed in the middle of the night, insisting that she had to get to the store. The more my aunt or I tried to convince her of the truth, the more insistent she became. It left all of us at our wits' end, crying and trying to keep her in the house. It was a nightmare.

I had read the Validation book a long time ago for some reason and then put it aside. Thank goodness I am a pack rat. I found it, and my aunt and I began to read it and tried to apply the techniques that are described. We both tried to enter my mother's world and tried to understand her need to work and feel productive again. Talking to my mother about the business, asking for her advice, and giving her old accounting journals seemed to help her. She carried these books under her arm and would go from room to room taking inventory, occasionally asking questions about a piece of furniture and making suggestions for difficult groupings. We are often rearranging the furniture to keep her calm; however, it is a small price to pay for the peace of mind that it seems to give my mother. Does it work all the time? No, sometimes she is just lost, but for the most part, it does.

WHY LYING, CONFRONTATION, AND PLAY-ACTING WILL NOT WORK

The Situation

Sarah's mother is expressing her need to be a productive person by trying to continue her daily work routine even though she is disoriented and has memory problems. She has moved into a personal reality in which she feels vital and has self-worth.

The Problem

Sara is grasping at various ways of coping with her mother's disoriented behavior, including playing along with the false beliefs, diverting her, and confronting her with reality. These methods sometimes work for short periods but often lead to more intense outbursts of anger or to withdrawal inward.

Lying for the good of the "patient" is sometimes called a *therapeutic lie*. However, disoriented and maloriented people are aware of reality on a preconscious level. It is simply that this reality is not helpful to them at the moment; either it is too painful to accept or it is not relevant or important. People who are in the final stage of life are often engaged with memories and the resolution of old, unfinished business. The here-and-now is not part of that process. If you pretend to believe that Sunday is really Monday, for example, then your mother will know on a subconscious level that you are pretending, and it will be difficult to have a trusting relationship. Build a relationship that is based on trust and love. From that, communication will flow.

There is a middle path between play-acting and confrontation: the acceptance of the personal reality that is expressed by the disoriented relative, with the knowledge that there is a very good reason behind it. Realize that it is not necessary to placate your mother to calm her down nor to "bring her back to reality." Try to explore the reason(s) behind her behavior and her beliefs. If you can fulfill the underlying need, then you can help her.

A Validation Approach

Step 1: Center yourself. Relax your body. Breathe deeply.

Step 2: Look at your mother. Match her emotion. Often, if you simply mirror the position of her mouth, chin, and eyes, you will capture the emotion and be able to have empathy.

Step 3: Explore what is going on in the moment. Forget what happened the last time you spoke with your mother, and do not worry about what will happen in the future. Stick to the present moment.

Sarah:	Hi Mom, what's going on?
Mother:	I've got to get to the store. We're late. What are you doing here?
Sarah:	I came to see how you're doing. How late are you?
Mother:	Well, you know we open at 10 A.M. What time is it?
Sarah:	Does it feel late to you?
Mother:	Everything is late.
Sarah:	You were always on time. Dad always said that if it weren't for you, the business would have failed. Where did you learn all that?
Mother:	From my mother. She always said that to be on time, you should be 10 minutes early. I taught you that. Al-

> ways be on time; keep your paperwork up to date and neat.
>
> Sarah: Mom, what did you enjoy the most about working in the store?
>
> Mother: I like to see the customers satisfied. You know I've had customers come in years after they bought something and say how happy they still are with their sofa.
>
> Sarah: A job well done, huh?
>
> Mother: Exactly.
>
> Sarah: What would happen if you couldn't work anymore?
>
> Mother: I would be lost. There'd be nothing left.
>
> Sarah: I see, work is everything that's important.
>
> Mother: That's right. If you don't work, you don't eat.
>
> Sarah: So it's important to keep on working.
>
> Mother: Right.
>
> Sarah: You have done a great job!
>
> Mother: Thanks, dear. You have, too.

When you are confronted with a direct question, such as, "What are you doing here?" it is important to take that seriously and answer it before exploring. It would not be respectful simply to ignore it. However, if you are asked a reality-based question that you suspect will be confronting if you answer it (e.g., "What time is it?"), then try to find a more exploratory way to respond. Often the topic of being late has a lot to do with feeling lost or left behind. It can be a more poetic way of saying, "I'm getting too old and life is passing me by."

You can move furniture, give her old accounting books, and ask your mother for advice, but be careful not to make it a game or play-act. What is most important is to take her need to be a productive, useful person seriously. This will help her feel more self-worth and fulfill the pressing need. Focus on showing your mother respect; value her lifetime of experience. She will definitely respond to that in a positive way, and you will be able enjoy your time with her.

✻

LOUISE AND TOM: LOSING YOUR HUSBAND

Tom and I have been married for a long time—36 years to be exact. I couldn't believe it when our doctor told us that Tom had Alzheimer's dementia. It was like someone kicked me in the gut. I can't imagine what it was like for him. My husband, Tom, is only 59 years old. We both joked a lot about his forgetfulness. Somewhere inside of me, I must have known it was more serious. Healthy people don't call you from the side of the road in a panic because they don't remember how to get to work, a route that Tom has traveled for 21 years. I must have known when he could not remember the names of our children when we went to dinner with a new business partner and his wife.

It's been hard to watch the changes in Tom. As a result of his declining ability to work, his company had to let him go. I was faced with a problem. After being home all those years taking care of our two children, I had to go back to work. Tom could be left alone at first, but later I found it hard to trust him. We tried adult day care, but the people there were so much older, it was awful. I got lucky; a retired neighbor, a man, comes and spends part of the day with Tom. They get along very well. I, on the other hand, struggle to talk with him and find it difficult just to be with him. He tells people that I have him locked up and have taken away all of his things. When I get home after a day of work, he starts with the same questions over and over: "Where are my keys?" "What have you done with my car?" He got so mad at me that he told me to leave his house. I kept telling myself, "This will get better," but it doesn't. Getting better means that Tom will have to get worse or, worse than that, die. I can't think about that, it makes me so sick; I wish I could throw the inside of me right out of me. If I cry, I will not stop!

A friend told me about a support group that she had heard about at one of our local retirement homes. Better than that, she went with me knowing that I would never go alone. It was interesting to hear what the others were talking about: Validation and how family members could use it. I began to listen, and some of the things that they were talking about began to make sense to me. I realized there that I had taken on the responsibility of making everything better. I had automatically believed that I had to make it better for him, for our kids, for everyone, even for me. The concept of freeing myself of the feeling that I had to "fix it" for Tom began to sink in. I realized that by trying to fix it, I was trying to be "in charge," to overcome the disease, but I can't make it go away. I can only learn to be with him in his pain or anger and be alright with it. That sounded like all I could do.

Several days later, I went with Tom to the gas station. It was awful! I could see that his ability to drive was quickly ending. He had a terrible time trying to get to the gas pumps. Nothing made sense to him. He began to get frustrated and angry. He got out of the car and started to shout and kick the car. People were looking. Even so, I got out of the car and tried to validate him. I rephrased the things he said, using the same voice tone and emotion. He began to calm down and look at me. Once we were back in the car, Tom began to cry and talked to me for the first time about how he was feeling. He told me how scared he gets; how awful it was not to be able to do the things that he had always done. I could ask him things such as, "When is it the worst?" "What is so scary?" "When aren't you scared?" Afterward, we both felt better. I think that he was relieved to tell me all that stuff. I didn't have to do anything. I listened and respected him. I had found a way to be with my husband, at least for now.

LOSING YOUR HUSBAND A LITTLE BIT EVERY DAY

The Situation

Early-onset Alzheimer's disease is more difficult to deal with than late onset. It is a degenerative process that cannot be cured; it keeps getting worse. It is particularly cruel in the beginning, when the person is acutely aware of the loss of cognitive function. It must be a little like watching your own body become paralyzed from the toes up. Watching your husband go through this and not being able to stop it is heartbreaking. You are called on to take on not only caring for your husband but also to become the primary wage earner in the family. It calls for extraordinary strength, flexibility, and courage.

The Problem

As Louise discovered, you cannot control the illness; you cannot prevent the decline. It is important to realize this and find a way of accepting the loss, a little bit at a time. Try not to deny the feelings of anger, frustration, pain, and sadness as they come up. Make room for them. Recognize that dealing with this takes a lot of energy. Do not be surprised when you find yourself tired more than usual.

A Validation Approach

Step 1: Center yourself; breathe and relax any tense muscles in your body. Remember that your goal is to find ways of communicating with your husband and to build a trusting, intimate relationship.

Step 2: Observe your husband; use matching and mirroring to find empathy.

Step 3: Listen to what your husband says, and explore the issues that seem important to him in that moment. Forget about what happened yesterday, and do not worry about what will happen tomorrow. Stay in the moment.

Tom:	What have you done with my car keys?
Louise:	When did you last have them?
Tom:	Yesterday. I put them right here in the key shell, and now they're gone.
Louise:	Are you missing anything else?
Tom:	Now that you mention it, my good pen is gone and my ID card for work.
Louise:	Do you mind if I give it a go and look?
Tom:	No, that would be great.
Louise:	(*looking through various suit jacket pockets*) It must drive you crazy to be missing all that stuff.
Tom:	You're not kidding. It seems that every time I put something down, it gets up and walks away.
Louise:	What do you miss the most?
Tom:	Going in everyday. Having a handle on things.
Louise:	You always prided yourself on handling things well. Do you remember when we had that car accident? Everyone was going nuts, but you were calm as can be.

Tom: Right. I called the police and then had everyone write down a statement so by the time the cops got there we were organized.

Louise: You were great.

Tom: Well, you're great too. What would I do without you now?

Louise: I love you, you know, no matter what.

    (*they hug*)

There are many different issues that Tom brings up. His sense of identity is tied to being organized and handling situations well. A car or car keys can be symbolic for manliness; if he often complains about missing his car, then he could be saying, "I miss being a man." That he is missing his work ID, his good pen, and his car would lead one to think that not being able to work was what was bothering him the most in the moment. He cannot work. That is the reality, but if Louise can find a way for him to handle situations or to remind him of ways that he did in the past so that he can re-live them, then it might help relieve his pain or frustration. By understanding the underlying meaning of Tom's words, Louise can perhaps have more empathy with him and find ways of addressing his need for identity, rather than the problem with the car keys.

Develop a support system for yourself, not just in terms of logistics (day care, household help, or community nursing), but also for your feelings. You might consider going to a support group for people in your situation. Your local Alzheimer Association is a good resource for finding what is available.

Try to find the positive moments of contact. These moments can be when you are reminiscing about the past or talking about his feelings in the moment. Sharing feelings can bring you closer; they are moments of intimacy and connection. Use empathy to connect to his feelings. A hug, a kiss, warm and loving eye contact, and an exchange of kind words are the little things that will help you both. Finding feelings of love for your husband will help lighten your load.

SOME FINAL THOUGHTS

Over and over, I have talked about focusing on the disoriented relative's needs and feelings and about putting your own needs and feelings aside. I'm sure that you are at the point of screaming, "Well what about me? What about my needs?" You cannot sublimate your own needs and feelings forever. Know this: Your needs are important; expressing your feelings is important. You have to take care of yourself and pay attention to your mental hygiene. Because your disoriented relative is unable to deal with your needs, it is important to find another place to do this.

Remember too that you cannot validate all day long. Choose your moments to listen actively and have empathy. The rest of the time, try to maintain a respectful, normal relationship.

Validation is not an answer for all disoriented elderly or their family members. It does not work in every situation. It is not a "magic bullet." However, if it does not work in one situation, then perhaps it will work in another. If you always validate from your heart, remaining respectful and caring, then Validation will never hurt either you or your relative. It is always worth trying.

Appendix 1

FAMILY MEMBER SUPPORT GROUP: COUNTRY MEADOWS, PENNSYLVANIA

Families who are struggling with the horror that Alzheimer's-related dementia inflicts quickly come to understand that this illness not only affects their loved one but also everyone who loves and cares for that person. These families begin a long and often painfully devastating journey of profound loss and suffering. When someone you love has dementia, it is like being shot in the heart. You often begin an emotional roller coaster ride of watching the light go out in someone for whom you care.

A Validation support group generally starts out in the same format as a Validation worker training course. Support group members are taught the same fundamentals, principles, theories, and techniques that are taught to Validation workers. It soon evolves into a tightly woven group, with a developing understanding and trust. Although lives and family situations are different, the feelings of profound loss, sadness, despair, anger, and rage are shared among everyone.

The support group focuses especially on the following six points:

- centering

- journaling

- role-playing

- acceptance ("you can't fix, and it's okay")

- empathy

- mentoring

Centering

For family members, centering exercises are critical. Feeling strong emotions has a tremendous impact on everyone's ability to be empathic; feelings that are evoked in family members can, for most, be a major obstacle. Centering exercises are taught and practiced routinely. Group members are encouraged and challenged to practice them daily. One critical point of centering is to help individuals not be "caught off guard." They develop the ability to be ready for whatever happens. This concept helps people to be ready to handle grief, sadness, anger, joy, love, and so forth. For example, one member's mother could be very passive and calm one minute, then, without warning, irritable and angry the next. She often accused the daughter of stealing her money and things. Before her daughter learned to center, her mother's words and actions embarrassed and hurt her daughter deeply. After learning centering exercises, she learned not to let the words get inside her but to work with her mother's anger over her losses.

Journaling

The concept of journaling—the fine art of committing pen to paper—is not anything new. It has been and continues to be a very effective tool to help get feelings out of that place that lies so deep in all of us. The act of writing can be an avenue to that interior place where pain and doubt linger. Group members are asked to keep a journal of their visits with their relative. They are asked to write about what happened, how they handled it, and which Validation techniques they used. Then, they are asked to identify the feelings that were stirred inside them in those situations. Writing about these feelings and situations gives individuals some distance and perspective on their feelings. Group members are encouraged to share their journal entries with fellow members. This generally leads to additional discussion, insights, and new perspectives.

Role-Playing

Role-playing, or acting out situations, becomes a critical means to re-create problematic situations and to gain a deeper understanding of the encounter. For most people, it is the first time they have ever had to "put on the skin" of someone else. Most have never taken on the thoughts and feelings of another person. Role-play allows them to experience someone's world through that person's eyes and ears. Many members report that role-playing, either watching or doing it, helped them to develop that "empathic sense." They were able to touch that raw feeling locked inside another person. Role-play also let many members experience the benefits of Validation techniques working and not working.

Acceptance ("You Can't Fix It, and It's Okay")

This concept is quite simple; it also is probably one of the hardest ideas for family members and practitioners of Validation to accept. We all have become brainwashed in the "fix it" mentality. We are truly conditioned to believe that something cannot be effective if someone or something is not changed in some positive way almost immediately. We all want that "look what I did" feeling. However, when family members begin to understand that old people are beyond the "fix me" mode, it opens them up to really doing some incredible things. It allows them to take in a person's needs, wants, dreams, hurts, fears, and so forth, without the need to generate a solution to change it or fix it. Sometimes the simplest thing is the most difficult to do. Success needs to be redefined as the ability to feel another person's soul for a moment and then bring closure to that moment with a smile, a song, a touch, a dance, or maybe just, "Can I come and talk with you again?" Success is the moment when you know that you have made a connection; you were part of that person's world.

Empathy

The ability to be empathic is not as easy as many may think. For family members, well, it may be easier to create life from a ball of clay. Often, years, decades, even centuries of "family stuff" can get in the way of all good intentions. It is an amazing phenomenon how old roles and rivalries that people had when they were younger once again emerge from the past to have an impact on their outlook and behavior as adults. Although helping family members develop an empathic ear can be challenging, it can be very rewarding. One of the first things that family members need to do is take off their judge and jury hats. They need to develop the understanding that empathy means not judging the needs, emotions, and reality of someone, but rather having the ability to experience them for what they are. For family members, the hard work begins when they begin to get in touch with all of their feelings that they have packed away. It is during this time that fellow group members are very helpful with insight, perspectives, and suggestions. When people realize that all families have their idiosyncrasies, they begin to realize that the "perfect family" exists only in television land. Just like older people, when family members can express their feelings and are actively listened to, the difficult feelings slowly lose power. Family members can grow comfortable in allowing the feelings of their loved ones to take up residence inside for just a little while. Understanding begins to grow instead of criticism. They develop the strength and the courage to begin the journey in someone else's shoes.

Mentoring

Of the numerous benefits to be generated from a Validation support group, one of the most beneficial is the birth of a mentor program for new family members. Mentors who are trained in Validation can be a tremendous influence to new members. Mentors act as both security blanket and confidant to help new members through the quagmire that comes with dementia. New family members can identify with a mentor because he or she is someone who has been through it. They share a common experience: loving someone with dementia. Mentors show new family members that there can be life beyond the painful moment. Mentors are living proof that this concept of Validation needs to be taken seriously. Mentors can be the person to whom families reach out for different thoughts, for answers to questions, and for other forms of support between group meetings. Mentors can help with the struggle of learning a new mindset while letting go of the old way of dealing with someone. Mentors can be the redefining difference in rebuilding those family bonds that are challenged by the inevitable process of growing old with dementia.

PROGRAMS OFFERED BY THE VALIDATION CENTER AT THE LANDESVEREIN FÜR INNERE MISSION IN DER PFALZ E.V.

In Germany, approximately 1.2 to 1.6 million people have some form of dementia; 80% of them remain in private homes. As a rule, people with dementia require a tremendous amount of care and attention, as well as supervision. In many cases, after a while, family caregivers find themselves on the boundaries of their endurance; they are exhausted and even become ill themselves. The Landesverein Für Innere Mission in der Pfalz E.V. (LVIM) has developed programs for family caregivers that offer information and training. These programs result in relief and a reduction of stress for both the caregiver and the disoriented family member, and make a difference in the quality of life at home.

The Hotline

The LVIM has set up a hotline telephone number to be able to answer the growing need for professional help in using a validating approach with disoriented very old people. Started in July 2004, the hotline enables professionals and nonprofessionals who work with disoriented very old family members or clients in the geographic area to call for advice in acute situations and get help from Certified Validation Practitioners.

House Visits

Certified Validation Practitioners, after talking in depth with family caregivers and gathering information, can go into a home situation and begin Validation contact with the very old person. This can be in everyday situations or in acute moments of stress. Additional visits can be arranged for continuing Validation at home. The situation is discussed with family caregivers, and guidance is given for a validating interaction with the disoriented very old relative.

The 3-Day Seminar for Family Caregivers

LVIM holds a 3-day seminar for people who are caring for disoriented very old people and who are open for new experiences in their relationship with them. The seminar includes the following:

- Introduction in the basic concepts of Validation
- Explanation of the reasons for disorientation in very old age
- The phases of resolution according to Naomi Feil
- Changing one's view of very old people
- Finding one's comfort zone
- Information on further training and available literature

Family Caregiver Training in Interaction

While the disoriented very old person is being validated by an experienced Certified Validation Practitioner in an adult care center or nursing facility, the family caregiver can be trained in Validation. Actual situations can be discussed and practiced with the seminar leader. The seminar leader (a certified Validation Teacher or Group Leader) can coach the family caregiver in her interactions with the disoriented relative. Both individual and group Validation are demonstrated during the seminar. Family caregivers learn coping strategies for their own personal daily situations and learn techniques that increase their sense of well-being.

FAMILY CAREGIVER COURSE IN VALIDATION

In several countries, Certified Validation Teachers offer special courses for family caregivers that concentrate on the practical elements of using Validation with disoriented older adults who live at home. It is recommended that all participants in this course attend a 1- or 2-day introductory workshop in Validation to gain a basic understanding of the method. This is followed by monthly meetings that last approximately 2 hours. The basic structure of each meeting is always the same:

- An opening round of greetings and making an inventory of issues to discuss later

- Practicing different ways of centering

- One topic to discuss and practice (with exercises if appropriate). Examples include how to look with validating eyes; finding an appropriate distance; what does not work: the difference between validation and diversion, lying, reality orientation, and other ways of coping; what is disorientation/dementia; important principles of Validation (that are practical and useful for family caregivers); and specific techniques that can be used at home.

- Coffee break
- Exchanging experiences and finding solutions to the problems presented at the beginning of the meeting

IN-HOME COUNSELING: AUSTRIAN MODEL

The Austrian Validation Organization has a list of Certified Validation Practitioners who are willing and able to assist family caregivers in their own home. A family caregiver can make direct contact with the Validation practitioner. The Validation practitioner can go into the home situation and have validating contact both in normal situations and in moments of crisis. This can be on an ongoing basis or limited. The situation is discussed with family caregivers, and guidance is given for a validating interaction with the disoriented very old relative.

These types of initiatives are crucial to family caregivers and should be encouraged in every country, in every state, and everywhere that disoriented elderly are being cared for by nonprofessionals at home. This relatively short summary of what is being done specifically for family caregivers should be seen as a source of inspiration as well as a source of support. It is hoped that this section of this book will expand and grow over time.

Appendix 2

Summary of Validation for Family Caregivers

Validation is a method for communicating with disoriented people who have received a diagnosis of some form of Alzheimer's-related dementia. It was developed by Naomi Feil, an American social worker, and first described in her book *Validation: The Feil Method*, published in 1982, and later in *The Validation Breakthrough: Simple Techniques for Communicating with People with "Alzheimer's-Type" Dementia*.

Validation does not try to make disoriented elderly people better, but rather gives caregivers the tools to change themselves so that they can enter the personal reality of the person for whom they are caring. Through a caring, empathic relationship, caregivers can reconnect or connect in a new way and give themselves and their disoriented relative more ease and pleasure.

Family members who care for disoriented loved ones are burdened with not only a physically challenging job, but also an emotional challenge on a large scale. Frustration, anger, sadness, pain, and loss can be daily experiences. If you have taken on this job, you can help yourself by

- Recognizing and respecting your own feelings
- Recognizing the feelings and needs of your disoriented relative, because these are distinctly different from your own
- Learning how to clear yourself of feelings, judgments, and worries for the short period of time when you want to validate
- Learning how to observe your relative carefully to pick up the clues that you need to explore her personal reality
- Developing a support system in which you can express your emotions, share your experiences, and get new ideas

Validation practitioners accept people just the way they are in the moment and do not try to change them. Your disoriented loved one cannot be expected to change and go "back to normal." The norm has changed. Acceptance is difficult because, in some ways, it means saying good-bye to the person whom you love.

Many family members think that it is better if the disoriented person is "brought back to reality." This is not always so. Think about what that means for your loved one: In the present reality, she has little worth, little to do to keep productive, and little authority or honor. There is nothing strongly holding your relative to the present reality and a great deal of pull from the past. The needs of elderly people are different from the needs of younger people. What you experience as important is not necessarily important to your relative. Other issues and other times of her life are perhaps more important. The person feels emotions that are leftover from her history. Things that have been bottled up over years come to the surface and demand attention. She expresses those feelings because it hurts to keep them inside. The best way to help your relative is to let her express whatever it is that needs to get out.

Malorientation, time confusion, repetitive motion, and vegetation are the four phases of resolution. They describe a process of retreating from the here and now, from the people around them, and from what is going on and the environment. It is a survival mechanism that is totally connected to a deep need to resolve, retreat, relive, and relieve. There is little in our reality that satisfies these needs. In fact, there is much in our reality that drives disoriented very old people to withdraw further. Following is a summary of how to validate:

- Center
- Observe
- Find the appropriate distance
- Find empathy

* Use the appropriate verbal techniques

  - Use open questions: who, what, where, when, or how
  - Rephrase what the person has said; use key words
  - Ask about the extreme
  - Reminisce about the past
  - Find a familiar coping mechanism
  - Use the preferred sense

* Use the appropriate nonverbal techniques

  - Mirroring
  - Genuine eye contact
  - Touch and anchored touch
  - Clear, warm voice tone
  - Observe, match, and say the emotion with emotion
  - Ambiguity
  - Link the behavior to the need
  - Music and singing

* End the conversation on a positive note

Appendix 3

CENTERING EXERCISES

The goal of each centering exercise is to reach a state of openness and resourcefulness. Clear away your thoughts and feelings, and make yourself ready to be empathic, to enter the world of the other person. Each of these exercises is a guided fantasy in which you use your imagination to change the state of your body and mind.

In all of the following exercises, you will stand or sit with your feet shoulder-width apart and feet flat on the floor. Make sure that you can feel the floor underneath your feet; if you are wearing shoes with heels, then take them off. Close your eyes. Breathe deeply from your belly in a relaxed way. Do not force the breaths. Mentally go through your body and relax your muscles, especially the places where you normally hold tension: shoulders, hands, face, stomach, and neck. When you feel relaxed and your breath is even and deep, you are ready to begin.

Centering with Color

Think of a color that gives you a good feeling. A feeling of strength, of openness, or of being able to handle whatever comes your way. Imagine that the air around you is this color, so every time you take in a breath of air you are taking this color into your body. Each time you inhale the color, it paints the inside of your body with this energy-giving color. As you exhale, the color spreads throughout the inside of your body, filling it with openness and a feeling of resourcefulness. With each breath, the color goes further. In your mind's eye, see the color spread through your torso, down your legs, into your feet, and into each toe.

With the next breath, follow the color through your shoulders, arms, and hands, and see it fill up each finger to the tips. With another breath, allow the color to fill your head. Now simply imagine the color, which is throughout your body, getting brighter with each breath you take. When you feel that the color is as strong as you can make it, come back to the here and now and open your eyes.

Centering with a Touch

Before beginning this exercise, choose a specific touch that you can use to "anchor" yourself. An anchor (in this context) is a connection between a mental state and a physical sensation, a bond, so that each time you do the touch, the mental state will be recalled. One anchor is to hold your right hand with your left hand so that the thumb is touching the inside of the palm, in the middle. Others are to cross your arms so that the fingers touch the elbows, or gently pinch an earlobe. Pick a touch that is special to you, one that you feel comfortable doing anywhere. The three images that follow show examples of different "touch anchors."

Once you have quieted yourself and are breathing evenly and deeply, imagine yourself in a situation in which you felt wonderful. Pick a situation that really happened, when you felt strong, open, and resourceful. You can handle anything that comes your way. You are at your best and most expansive. Really picture the

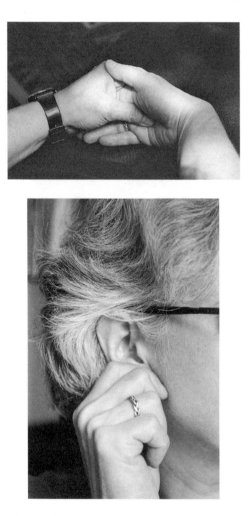

situation and what happened. See the environment around you, hear the sounds, and feel them as well. Is it warm there or cool? Is the wind rushing, or can you sense the silence? Feel how open your heart is. When this feeling is at its strongest, do the touch that you have chosen and hold it with some pressure for a count of 10, then relax in that same position. When you feel ready, come back to the present and open your eyes.

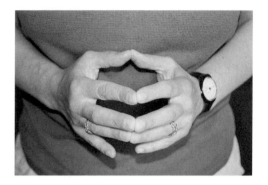

Centering with Sound

Think of a sound or a piece of music that gives you a feeling of expansiveness, of strength, and of opening yourself to your resources. It could be a voice, a sound from nature, or a special piece of music. Hear this sound in your imagination. Imagine the sound; tune into it and the feelings that it stimulates. Hear how it resonates in your body. Harmonize with the sound. Sense the strength that comes from within you and feel yourself opening to new possibilities. You are becoming ready to handle whatever comes your way. You are clear. When you are ready, come back to the present and open your eyes.

Each exercise is connected with a preferred sense: visual, kinesthetic, or auditory. Pick the one that resonates with you the best, and practice it every day for approximately 5 minutes. You will find that after a week or so, it will become easier to do; you will be able to center yourself and feel resourceful quickly. This can be very useful in your day-to-day life, when you need to deal with stressful situations of any nature.

Appendix 4

VALIDATION AND ALZHEIMER'S DISEASE INFORMATION RESOURCES

Web Sites

www.vfvalidation.org

www.validation-eva.com

Authorized Validation Organizations

Contact in the United States

George M. Leader Institute
Jana Stoddard
830 Cherry Drive
Hershey, PA 17033, USA

Phone: 717-533-2474
Fax: 717-533-6202
E-mail: Jstoddard@countrymeadows.com

Austria

For Vienna, Lower Austria, and Burgenland:
Validation Academy
Ausbildungszentrum des Wiener Roten Kreuzes
Franzosengraben 8
A-1030 Vienna, Austria
Phone: 43-1-79580-6302
Fax: 43-1-79580-9600
E-mail: validation@w.redcross.or.at

For Upper Austria, Salzburg, and Steirmark:
Ulrike Praschl
Samariterbund Linz
Reindlstraße 24
4040 Linz, Austria
Phone: 43-732-736466-0
E-mail: avo@asb.or.at

Belgium

Didier Barbieux
Rhapsodie
Chaussée de Waterloo 788
1180 Brussels, Belgium
Phone: 32-2-372-2351
Fax: 32-2-372-2332
E-mail: rhapsodie@skynet.be

France

Association pour la promotion de la Validation Therapy
M.Y. Georges, President
Phone/Fax: 33-383-27-83-16
Cell: 33-6-84-85-88-56
E-mail: sec.apvapa@wanadoo.fr

Insitut de formation M&R
Kathia Munsch
5, rue des 3 Piliers
51100 Reims, France
Phone/Fax: 03-26-87-20-88
E-mail: kathia.munsch@wanadoo.fr

Germany

For Saarland, Rheinland-Pfalz, Hessen, Thuringen:
Hedwig Neu
Landesverein für Innere Mission in der Pfalz
Dr. Kaufmann Strasse 2
67098 Bad Dürkheim, Germany
Phone: 49-6322-607-230
Fax: 49-6322-607-103
E-mail: validation@lvim-pfalz.de

For Baden Württemberg, Bayern, Nordrhein-Westfalen:
Wolfgang Hahl
Mannheimer Akademie
Deutsches Rotes Kreuz
Heinrich-Lanz-Strasse 5
68165 Mannheim, Germany
Phone: 49-621-833-7040
Fax: 49-621-833-7049
E-mail: wolfgang.hahl@mannheimer-akademie.de

For Niedersachsen, Sachsen, Schleswig Holstein, Bremen,
    Hamburg:
Heidrun Tegeler
Paritätische Gesellschaft für soziale Dienste, Bremen mbH
Dienstleistungszentrum Vegesack
Zum Alten Speicher 10
28759 Bremen, Germany
Phone: 49-421-66-24-99
Fax: 49-421-27-70-941
E-mail: h.tegeler@paritaet-bremen.de

For Brandenburg, Mecklenburg-Vorpommern, Berlin:
Thomas Schelzky
Insitut für Angewandte Gerontologie
Haubachstrasse 8
10585 Berlin, Germany
Phone: 49-30-341-5034
Fax: 49-30-341-6068
E-mail: thomas.schelzky@ifag-berlin.de

Switzerland

Tertianum AG, ZfP
Seestrasse 110
CH-8267 Berlingen, Switzerland
Phone: 41-52-762-5757
Fax: 41-52-762-5770
E-mail: c.niebergall@tertianum.ch

Sweden

Kristina Telerud
Ersta diakonisällskap
Erstagatan 1
116 91 Stockholm, Sweden
Phone: 46-8-714-6217
Fax: 46-8-714-6673
E-mail: kristina.telerud@ersta.se

European Manager

Vicki de Klerk-Rubin
E-mail: vdeklerk@vfvalidation.org

ALZHEIMER'S DISEASE–RELATED RESOURCES

Web Sites

www.alz.org

This site is especially for family members and offers many possibilities for support information and groups.

www.mayoclinic.com

This site offers good articles and medical information.

www.alzheimersupport.com

This site offers a chat room where members can offer each other support.

References

Alzheimer, A., & Nissl, F. (1904–1918). *Histologic and histopathologic studies of the cerebral cortex* (6 Vols.). Jena, Germany: G. Fisher.

American Psychiatric Association. (1994). *Diagnostic and statistical manual of mental disorders (4th ed.).* Washington, DC: American Psychiatric Association.

Atkinson, R. L., Atkinson, C. R., Smith, E. E., & Bem, D. J. (1993). *Introduction to Psychology.* (11th ed.). Fort Worth, TX: Harcourt Brace Jovanovich.

Feil, N. (1982, 2003). *V/F Validation: The Feil method.* Cleveland, OH: Edward Feil Productions.

Feil, N. (2002). *The Validation breakthrough: Simple techniques for communicating with people with "Alzheimer's-type dementia."* Baltimore: Health Professions Press.

Folstein, M., Folstein, S., & McHugh, P. *Mini-Mental State Examination (MMSE).* Lutz, FL: Psychological Assessment Resources. Available at www.parinc.com.

Merriam-Webster, A. (1980). *Webster's New Collegiate Dictionary.* Springfield, MA: G & C Merriam Co.

National Center for Health Statistics. Available at www.cdc.gov (table 27, Life Expectancy at Birth).

Van Diemen, R., & van de Niewegiessen, C. (1995). Met een been aan de andere Kant, Nijkerk, The Netherlands: Intro Publishers.

World Health Organization. (1992). *The ICD-10 classification of mental and behavioural disorders.* Geneva: World Health Organization.

Index

Note: Page numbers followed by *b* indicate boxes, those followed by *f* indicate figures, those followed by *p* indicate photos, those followed by *t* indicate tables.

overview of, 6–9, 8*f*
resources on, 121
See also Alzheimer's disease
Dementia of the Alzheimer's
Type (DAT) with late
onset, 12–14, 13*b*. *See also*
Disoriented old-old
Disorientation
appropriate distance with, 65
coping and, 37–38
reality and, 16, 20, 23
from strokes, 9–10
Validation theory on, 14
See also Malorientation phase;
Time confusion phase
Disoriented old-old
acceptance of, 16–17, 18–19
Dementia of the Alzheimer's
Type (DAT) and, 13, 13*b*
feelings of (*See* Feelings of
disoriented old-old)
meaning of behavior of (*See*
Meaning of behavior)
needs of, 25–30, 57, 59–60,
67–68
valuing, 17–18, 18*b*, 95
Distance appropriate for
communication, 45–46,
65. *See also* Validation:
case studies
Dos and don'ts for youth/
children, 80
Drugs. *See* Medications

Emergencies and disorientation,
9
Emotions. *See* Feelings of disoriented old-old; Feelings of
family members
Empathy
definition of, 39

example in case study, 68
finding, 46, 104
meaning of behavior and, 99
role-playing and, 103
trust building and, 25
Eye contact, establishing, 52

Families
acceptance and, 16–17
coping of, 14–17, 23
feelings of (*See* Feelings of
family members)
self-care of: needs and feelings, 100, 110*b*; positive
moments, 99; respecting
own limits, 60–61; steps
in, 15–16, 17, 110*b*
stress of, 74–75
support for (*See* Support for
families)
Validation training for, 3, 61,
105–108
Family Member Support Group
(Country Meadows, PA),
101–105
Father/child relationship. *See*
Parent/child relationship
Father-touch, 52, 53*p*, 55
Feelings of disoriented old-old
anchored touch and, 52, 53*p*,
54*p*, 55, 55*p*
being at home and, 89–90
expression of, 23–24, 27, 75
in malorientation case study,
72
needs and, 60
nonverbal communication
and, 55, 56–58
recognizing from nonverbal
cues, 42, 43*p*, 44*p*, 45*p*
sexuality and, 26

acceptance and, 18–20
concerns with lateness, 95
empathy and, 99
needs unmet and, 25–30, 57
repeated questions, 67–68
stealing accusations, 78, 80
Medications
as chemical restraints, 27
disorientation and, 9–10
sensory functioning and, 26
Memory
balance in life and retrieval
of, 21
forgetting family members,
75, 84–85
of past vs. reality, 23
repetition of questions, 66,
69
sensory, 21–22
See also Reminiscing
Mentoring, 105
Mini-Mental State Examination,
12
Mirroring technique, 52
Mother/child relationship. *See*
Parent/child relationship
Mothering vs. nurturing, 26
Mother-touch, 52, 53*p*, 55
Music
centering with, 116
as communication, 58, 77,
82, 84

Needs of disoriented old-old
feelings of self-worth and, 60
meaning of behavior and,
25–30, 57
repetitive questions and,
67–68
sensory stimulation and, 59
See also Meaning of behavior

Neurons in Alzheimer's disease,
7, 8*f*
Nonverbal communication
techniques
feelings of disoriented old-old
and, 55, 56–58
summary of, 58*b*, 112*b*
touch, 46, 52, 53*p*, 54*p*, 55,
55*p*, 88
See also Validation: case studies; Verbal communication
techniques
Not being recognized, 75, 84–88
Nurturing vs. mothering, 26

Observing
overview of, 41–42, 43*p*, 44*p*,
45*p*, 64–65
youth and, 79
See also Validation: case
studies
Old-old. *See* Disoriented old-old
Open questions. See under
Questions

Parent/child relationship
acceptance in, 16–17, 81–84
case studies: acceptance,
81–84; lying and
play-acting, 92–95;
malorientation, 71–74;
repeating questions,
65–68; respecting the
adult, 74–77; time
confusion, 68–71
examples, 31–32, 33–34
touch and, 52, 53*p*, 55
Partner-touch, 52, 54*p*, 55. *See
also* Husband/wife
relationship
Physical exams, 11–12